Millie Boettcher, RN, MSN
Ped. Clinical Nurse Specialist

ESOPHAGEAL MOTILITY TESTING

ESOPHAGEAL MOTILITY TESTING

Editors

Donald O. Castell, MD, FACP

Chief, Gastroenterology Section
Professor of Medicine
Bowman Gray School of Medicine
Winston-Salem, North Carolina

Joel E. Richter, MD, FACP

Associate Professor of Medicine
Bowman Gray School of Medicine
Winston-Salem, North Carolina

Christine Boag Dalton, PA-C

Physicians Assistant
Gastroenterology Division
Bowman Gray School of Medicine
Winston-Salem, North Carolina

Elsevier
New York · Amsterdam · London

Elsevier Science Publishing Co., Inc.
52 Vanderbilt Avenue, New York, New York 10017

Distributors outside the United States and Canada:

Elsevier Science Publishers B.V.
P.O. Box 211, 1000 AE Amsterdam, the Netherlands

Library of Congress Cataloging in Publication Data

Esophageal motility testing.
Includes index.
1. Esophagus — Motility — Disorders — Diagnosis.
2. Esophagus — Motility — Measurement. I. Castell,
Donald O. II. Richter, Joel E. III. Dalton, Christine
Boag. [DNLM: 1. Esophageal Diseases — diagnosis.
2. Esophagus — physiology. 3. Gastrointestinal Motility.
4. Manometry — methods. WI 250 E7653]
RC815.7.E755   1987   616.3′20754   Pms.87-13517

ISBN 0-444-01244-3

Current printing (last digit):
10 9 8 7 6 5 4 3 2

Manufactured in the United States of America

Contents

Preface / ix
Acknowledgments / xi
Contributors / xiii

PART I
ESTABLISHING THE LABORATORY

1. **Historical Perspectives and Current Use of Esophageal Manometry** / 3
   Donald Castell, MD, FACP
   Historical Perspective / 3
   Conclusion / 11

2. **Anatomy and Physiology of the Esophagus and Its Sphincters** / 13
   Donald O. Castell, MD, FACP
   Anatomy / 13
   Physiology / 14

3. **The Esophageal Motility Laboratory: Materials and Equipment** / 28
   Christine Boag Dalton, PA-C
   Primary Equipment / 28
   Secondary Equipment / 33

4. The Manometric Study / 35
Christine Boag Dalton, PA-C
Preparation for the Study / 35
Intubation / 37
The Manometric Study / 39
The Lower Esophageal Sphincter / 42
The Body of the Esophagus / 48
Provocative Testing / 56
Upper Esophageal Sphincter / 57

5. Measurements and Interpretations / 61
Christine Boag Dalton, PA-C
Lower Esophageal Sphincter Pressure / 61
Upper Esophageal Sphincter / 76
Final Report / 78

6. Normal Values for Esophageal Manometry / 79
Joel E. Richter, MD, FACP
Prior Studies / 79
Normal Values Based on Our Experience in 95 Healthy Volunteers / 80
Conclusion / 89

7. The Computer in the Motility Laboratory / 91
June A. Castell, MS
Introduction / 91

PART II
ABNORMAL ESOPHAGEAL MOTILITY

8. Achalasia / 107
Philip O. Katz, MD
Clinical Presentation / 107
Radiologic Features / 108
Endoscopy / 108
Manometry / 109
Lower Esophageal Sphincter / 109
Esophageal Body / 110
Atypical Findings / 112
Treatment / 115

9. Diffuse Esophageal Spasm / 118
Joel E. Richter, MD, FACP
Historical Background / 118
Pathophysiology and Etiology / 119
Symptoms / 119
Manometric Diagnosis / 121
Conclusions / 128

10. The Nutcracker Esophagus and Other Primary Esophageal Motility Disorders / 130
Donald O. Castell, MD, FACP
Nutcracker Esophagus / 131
The Hypertensive Lower Esophageal Sphincter / 138
Nonspecific Esophageal Motility Disorders / 139

11. Noncardiac Chest Pain: Use of Esophageal Manometry and Provocative Tests / 143
Joel E. Richter, MD, FACP
Initial Evaluation: Rule out Heart Disease / 144
Esophageal Testing / 144
Esophageal Manometry / 145
Provocative Tests / 146
Future Developments / 151

12. Exogenous Factors Affecting Esophageal Motility / 156
Thomas P. McMahon, MD
Tobacco-Containing Products / 156
Alcohol / 157
Food / 158
Temperature / 159

13. Secondary Motility Disorders / 163
Martin W. Scobey, MD
Introduction / 163
Collagen-Vascular Diseases / 164
Endocrine and Metabolic Disorders / 168
Neuromuscular Disorders / 172
Chronic Idiopathic Intestinal Pseudo-Obstruction / 176
Chagas' Disease / 178
Aging and the Esophagus / 178

14. The Upper Esophageal Sphincter / 183
W.E. Roger Green, MB, FRCS (England), MS (London) and Donald O. Castell, MD, FACP
Upper Esophageal Sphincter Pressures / 184
The Hypopharynx / 184
Coordination of Hypopharynx and the Upper Esophageal Sphincter / 185
Manometry of the Pharyngoesophageal Junction / 190
Protocol for Upper Esophageal Sphincter Manometry / 192
Analysis of the Manometry Record / 192
Assessment of Upper Esophageal Sphincter Manometry Data / 192
Disorders of the Upper Esophageal Sphincter / 193

15. Gastroesophageal Reflux and pH Testing / 198
Wallace C. Wu, MB, BS
Esophageal Manometry / 198
Intraesophageal pH Measurements / 199

Index / 209

Preface

During the past 20 years there has been a greater interest in human esophageal motility, including both normal function and abnormalities that produce clinical syndromes. This has resulted in a remarkable increase in the numbers of esophageal motility laboratories throughout the United States established for the purposes of either performing clinical studies in symptomatic patients or for investigation of esophageal function. To date, there has been little specific information provided on how to establish an esophageal motility laboratory, how to perform a satisfactory and useful manometric study, and how to interpret some of the motility findings in symptomatic patients. Our experience over the last 20 years has included hundreds of studies on patients and a vast array of pharmacologic and physiologic tests in normal volunteers. The purpose of this text is to bring together this experience in an attempt to describe the mechanisms by which modern techniques can be applied to the study of normal and abnormal esophageal motility and to suggest criteria for interpretation for manometric findings.

Our experience with esophageal motility testing, both in the clinical arena and as a research tool, is quite extensive and has allowed us to develop many concepts and beliefs concerning the proper application of the esophageal motility laboratory to clinical medicine. In the final analysis, then, this work represents a fairly complete statement of our concepts of esophageal motility testing, which includes discussions of the bases for the things that we do, the methods by which they are accomplished, the rationale for the interpretation of data, and the clinical application of the tests results. It is our sincere hope that the reader will find this text of considerable value in the practice of this art and will find sufficient solid justification for the approaches discussed in this text — that esophageal motility can be considered to have become a science.

Acknowledgments

The authors wish to express their sincere appreciation to the members of the Medicine Satellite Center (Linda Brown, Karen Chatman, and Tammy Allgood) for their support, by typing the many chapters of this book. We acknowledge the support of our many colleagues who have helped us develop our current concepts of esophageal motility testing over the years. Finally, we wish to express our gratitude to Ms. Rebecca Southard for her diligent and valuable assistance in organizing and preparing this text.

Contributors

Donald O. Castell, MD, FACP
Chief, Gastroenterology Section; Professor of Medicine, Bowman Gray School of Medicine, Winston-Salem, North Carolina

June A. Castell, MS
Computer Analyst, Gastroenterology Division, Bowman Gray School of Medicine, Winston-Salem, North Carolina

Christine Boag Dalton, PA-C
Physicians Assistant, Gastroenterology Division, Bowman Gray School of Medicine, Winston-Salem, North Carolina

W.E. Roger Green, MB, FRCS (England), MS (London)
Formerly Surgical Research Consultant, Gastroenterology Division, Bowman Gray School of Medicine, Winston-Salem, North Carolina

Philip O. Katz, MD
Assistant Professor of Medicine, Gastroenterology Division, Francis Scott Key Medical Center, Baltimore, Maryland

Thomas P. McMahon, MD
Gastroenterology Division, Aquidneck Medical Center, Newport, Rhode Island

Joel E. Richter, MD, FACP
Associate Professor of Medicine, Bowman Gray School of Medicine, Winston-Salem, North Carolina

Martin W. Scobey, MD
Fellow, Gastroenterology Division, Bowman Gray School of Medicine, Winston-Salem, North Carolina

Wallace C. Wu, MB, BS
Professor of Medicine, Bowman Gray School of Medicine, Winston-Salem, North Carolina

ESOPHAGEAL MOTILITY TESTING

PART I

ESTABLISHING
THE LABORATORY

Historical Perspectives and Current Use of Esophageal Manometry

Donald O. Castell, MD, FACP

During the past decade, there has been a remarkable resurgence of interest in studies of esophageal function. Improvements in methodology for accurate measurement of intraluminal pressures with greater sophistication of studies of the lower esophageal sphincter (LES) began this reawakening, and it continued through the more recent refinements in the measurement of esophageal peristaltic pressures and, finally, upper esophageal sphincter evaluation. In addition, initial studies showing that large amounts of gastrin could increase LES pressure opened the door to a whole series of investigations of the effects of hormones and, more recently, the effects of a variety of other possible pharmacologic agents on esophageal function. It is my intention to provide perspective, to attempt to identify the studies that have led to the current "truths" of esophageal manometrics, and to assess their importance in the clinical practice of medicine.

HISTORICAL PERSPECTIVE

Manometric studies were first performed by Kronecker and Meltzer in 1883[1] and Meltzer in 1894[2] using air-filled balloons and an external pressure transducer. Water-filled balloons were first used by Ingelfinger and Abbot in 1940.[3] Because of their inaccuracy and delayed assessment of rapid pressure changes in the esophagus, these methods were not found clinically useful and were abandoned.

Studies with water-filled catheters first began in the 1950s and initiated development of the basic knowledge of the physiology and pathophysiology of esophageal motility. The LES was first identified manometrically by Fyke et al in 1956.[4]

Techniques

The choice of a method for measurement of esophageal pressures resides with the use of either a water-filled catheter connected to external transducers or a catheter assembly containing small direct intraluminal transducers. The studies of Pope[5] and Harris and Winans[6] led to the replacement of static water-filled catheters within the esophagus by systems employing constant infusion of small quantities of water. They found that the true recording of magnitude of squeeze exerted on a catheter orifice by a tonic sphincter required sufficient infusion of fluid within the catheter to overcome the "yield pressure" exerted by the sphincter.[1] Using these newer perfusion techniques, Cohen and Harris showed in subsequent studies excellent correlation between the LES pressure measurement and the assessment of LES strength. The latter was estimated by recording the force required to pull a 1-cm Teflon ball through the LES.[8] Although very slow infusion rates are required (less than 1.0 mL/min) to record tonic sphincter squeeze, later studies indicated that a more vigorous infusion rate within the catheter was required to record accurately the rapidly changing transient high pressures produced during intraesophageal peristaltic activity.[9,10] Refinements in technology made it apparent that decreasing the degree of compliance within the catheter system by eliminating syringes in the infusion set-up and using small rigid tubing would allow accurate measurement of rapid transient changes in intraesophageal pressure without the necessity of high infusion rates.[11] At present, the preferred system of fluid-filled catheter manometry should include a pneumohydraulic infusion pump and small (0.8-mm internal diameter) polyvinyl tubing. The choice of external pressure transducers and recording systems can be left to the user.

Accurate recording of sphincter pressure and esophageal peristaltic pressures can also be obtained with small direct intraluminal transducers. A comparison of this technique with the best infusion techniques reveals excellent correlation.[9,10] Many clinical motility laboratories are equipped with methodology of this kind; the resulting lack of dependence on infusion pumps and fluid-filled systems is considered an asset. A major drawback of this system is its nonavailability when any of these small transducers are malfunctioning, as the entire assembly must be returned to the factory for repair. In addition, the fixed position of the transducers in the catheter assembly does not allow flexibility of change in design for location of pressure recording sites in experimental studies. Either system, however, is satisfactory for quantitative clinical studies when properly applied.

Lower Esophageal Sphincter Pressure Measurement

The method of recording LES pressure and its clinical relevance have been subjects of considerable controversy. Most reported manometric studies have recorded LES pressure by slowly withdrawing a catheter orifice from stomach to esophagus across the high-pressure zone generated by the sphincter. The usual technique involves moving the catheter in 0.5- to 1.0-cm increments, leaving it "stationed" at each level for a few seconds before advancing further (the "station pull-through" technique). A modification of this technique involves having the patient suspend respiration while the catheter orifice is in the stomach and then rapidly withdrawing the catheter orifice across the LES into the esophagus before respiration is resumed (the "rapid pull-through" technique). The first quantitative recording of LES pressure using the rapid pull-through (RPT) technique was done in 1972 by Waldeck.[12] This technique was subsequently refined by Dodds et al.[13] With either of these techniques, the LES pressure is measured as the gradient between gastric pressure and maximal pressure within the sphincter. Similar results are obtained when the two techniques are compared in the same patient at the same sitting, with the RPT technique consistently providing values 2–3 mm Hg higher than the station pull-through (SPT) technique. It seems to matter little whether the SPT or RPT technique is utilized to measure resting LES pressure, so this decision may also be left to the user. However, LES relaxation in response to swallowing can only be assessed with the catheter stationed in the LES.

An important question has arisen concerning the clinical relevance of an isolated LES pressure. This question is compounded by the observation that pressures recorded in various directions within the sphincter are not equal[14] and that pressures recorded in the same sphincter of the same individual at different periods of time and after various physiologic changes (meals, position, etc) vary considerably. Thus, it becomes quite difficult to decide which sphincter pressure is the "true" pressure and what the significance of a basal LES pressure is in the clinical interpretation of esophageal function. A rational approach to this problem has been to pull a series of three to eight recording orifices across the LES and to utilize a mean value as the LES pressure. Perhaps it would be even more rational to use the highest (or even the lowest) pressure measured during any one study. Recent studies in cats have suggested that the end-expiratory pressure represents a true measurement of sphincter pressure.[15] The recently developed Dent sleeve offers the advantage of a longer (6 cm) segment of the recording catheter for better positioning in prolonged monitoring of LES pressure.[16] This is primarily a research tool to be used in studies of pressure changes over long periods.

Initial studies suggested that LES pressure measurements might have value in separating the patient with a strong potential for gastroesophageal reflux from the nonrefluxing patient.[6] Subsequent experience revealed considerable overlap between sphincter pressures in these two patient groups, resulting in much disillusionment about the clinical usefulness of this test.[17] Although a normal LES pressure range is usually between 10 and 45 mm Hg in most laboratories, it is only at the extremes that the measurement has diagnostic value. Thus, a sphincter pressure of less than 6 mm Hg gives fairly reliable predictability of the potential for reflux.

Intraesophageal Peristaltic Pressure Measurement

Improvements in infusion methods and the use of direct intraluminal transducers have generated new concepts of normal and abnormal peristaltic pressures. High-amplitude esophageal contractions were once considered to be identified by any pressures greater than 40 mm Hg. With modern techniques, it is now known that average normal amplitude in the distal esophagus is approximately 100 mm Hg and that isolated peristaltic contraction pressures of up to 200 mm Hg should not be considered abnormal.[9] In addition, other aspects of the normal peristaltic sequence, such as the frequency or absence of a peristaltic response to a swallow and the velocity and duration of a contraction wave, have been more critically evaluated. It has become apparent that reproducible and accurate quantitative assessment of the peristaltic sequence involves not only the use of an appropriate recording system, but also the afferent stimulation by a liquid bolus in the pharynx (a "wet swallow").[18,19] When evaluating esophageal peristaltic activity in our laboratory, we routinely perform a series of "wet swallows" (3- to 5-mL water bolus), usually separated by a 20- to 30-sec interval to allow the esophagus to return to a stable baseline. Manometric studies performed in this fashion provide the opportunity for more specific quantitative assessment of esophageal squeeze and should be part of all clinical esophageal motility studies.

Use of Esophageal Manometry

In recent times, there has been considerable controversy over the accuracy, reproducibility, and importance of pressures measured in the esophagus and its sphincters. This has led to confusion about the potential clinical utility of esophageal manometry in the diagnosis of abnormalities of esophageal function. There are at least two important aspects that should be considered when formulating an opinion concerning the clinical utility of manometry. The first aspect relates to the frequent use of esophageal manometry in both the clinical and the basic research laboratory. There has been widespread use of manometric techniques to study pharmacophysiology of the esophagus in health and disease. Studies performed in a variety of species, including humans, primates, cats, dogs, and opossums, have provided much new information on esophageal function. One should keep in mind, therefore, that a major use of esophageal manometry is in the research environment for the purpose of understanding both normal function and disease. It is important not to confuse this aspect of esophageal manometry with the question of its clinical utility.

A second important aspect in the current development of esophageal manometric testing relates to the vastly improved technology presently available. With the development of direct intraluminal transducers and low-compliance infusion systems, it is now possible to perform more precise and quantitative measurements of abnormal esophageal pressures. These developments clearly promise the prospect of greater clinical utility for esophageal manometry. It is important to recognize that much of the older literature provides values for esophageal pressure measurements recorded with highly compliant infusion systems, which make measurements of contractile amplitude of the peristaltic wave grossly inaccurate. One should also recognize the importance of studying patients only in manometric laboratories that employ the best techniques available at the present time.

Clinical Application of Esophageal Manometric Studies

The major value of an esophageal manometry laboratory in clinical practice is in the diagnosis of esophageal motility dysfunction. These conditions can be subdivided into two types: those in which the motility defect is a primary condition involving only the esophagus and those in which an esophageal abnormality is a secondary aspect of a more generalized disease. The physician utilizing the esophageal manometric laboratory for diagnostic help should recognize these distinctions and note particularly the potential for esophageal motility disorders in various systemic diseases.

Those entities in which motility changes are almost pathognomonic include scleroderma and achalasia. These are described in detail in Chapters 8 and 13. The important manometric feature of sclerodermatous involvement of the esophagus is the marked abnormality in the smooth muscle portion of this organ (lower two-thirds) with relative normalcy of the striated muscle segment (upper one-third). Similarly, achalasia in its classic form is also well defined by specific manometric criteria characterized primarily by a poorly relaxing, hypertensive LES and total absence of esophageal peristalsis.

For the clinician, the paramount problem is to define the real value of esophageal manometry in more precise diagnosis of patients with symptoms potentially of esophageal origin (Table 1.1).

Dysphagia

There are few who would argue that esophageal manometry is useful in evaluating the patient with dysphagia, for this is often the means by which a specific diagnosis of certain esophageal motility abnormalities can be made. This may apply specifically to scleroderma, achalasia, and diffuse esophageal spasm and its variants. In our laboratory more than 50% of patients with a presenting complaint of dysphagia will have abnormal motility.

In approaching the patient with dysphagia, however, it is not my contention that esophageal manometry is always necessary or that it should be included as an initial diagnostic approach. I would suggest that the barium esophagram be the initial diagnostic screening test in patients with dysphagia. If this test reveals an apparent mechanical obstructing lesion (stricture,

TABLE 1.1 Suggested Clinical Uses of Esophageal Motility Testing

Evaluation of patients with dysphagia
  Primary esophageal motility disorders
    Achalasia
    Diffuse esophageal spasm
    Hypertensive LES
    Nutcracker esophagus
    Nonspecific esophageal motility disorders
  Secondary esophageal motility disorders
    Scleroderma

Evaluation of patients with possible gastroesophageal reflux disease
  Support diagnosis in a complex patient
    Atypical symptoms
    Failed medical therapy
  Evaluate defective peristalsis (particularly prior to fundoplication)
  Exclude scleroderma
  Assist in placement of pH probe

Evaluation of patients with noncardiac chest pain
  Primary esophageal motility disorders
  Pain response to provocative testing

Exclude generalized gastrointestinal tract disease
  Scleroderma
  Chronic idiopathic intestinal pseudo-obstruction

Exclude esophageal etiology for suspected anorexia nervosa

carcinoma, ring), then esophagoscopy is usually the next most appropriate, and often final, diagnostic test. However, if the esophagram fails to reveal a definite abnormality or apparent mechanical obstruction, manometric testing then becomes the next preferred diagnostic procedure.

Gastroesophageal Reflux

Motility studies have little use in the routine evaluation of patients with symptomatic gastroesophageal (GE) reflux. There are, however, some situations in which these studies may be of value. One example is the patient with atypical symptoms or in whom antireflux medical therapy is ineffective.

Sphincter pressures can be assessed and, if they are very low (< 6 mm Hg), a diagnosis of reflux can be supported. Manometry will also give information regarding peristaltic function and will aid in optimal placement of pH probe for intraesophageal pH testing, if it is desired.

Patients with suspected scleroderma are another group in whom manometry may prove useful for evaluation of reflux. Esophageal involvement is frequent (70%–80%) in these patients and symptoms may be misleading despite very low LES pressure and decreased amplitude of peristalsis in the lower esophagus.[20] Manometry may help confirm the diagnosis if the combination of very low LES pressure and weak-to-absent peristalsis in the distal esophagus is found. This manometric pattern becomes almost pathognomonic for scleroderma when found in combination with a normal upper esophageal sphincter pressure and normal upper esophageal peristalsis.

It is our feeling that all patients being considered for antireflux surgery should be evaluated manometrically. An alternative diagnosis can rarely be made. More importantly, preoperative manometry allows assessment of the adequacy of peristaltic pressures in the esophageal body. If the patient has a severely disordered or weak peristalsis, a fundoplication may result in postoperative dysphagia, due to defective esophageal clearing. With the preoperative information of weak peristalsis, the surgeon may wish to perform a "loose" fundoplication or to postpone surgery until another trial of medical therapy can be completed.

At present, the major value for the manometry laboratory in GE reflux appears to be in research. Work in the last 20 years has provided much insight into the pathogenesis of reflux disease and has allowed evaluation of pharmacologic and environmental agents as causes of reflux, as well as investigation of numerous therapeutic modalities.

Noncardiac Chest Pain

There is increasing awareness of the potential application of esophageal manometry in the evaluation of patients with chest pain, particularly those in whom cardiac disease has been carefully excluded. At the present time, chest pain is the major reason for referral of patients to most active esophageal manometry laboratories. It is too soon to make a final statement on the true utility and effectiveness of manometry in the evaluation of this subset of patients. Unquestionably, a specific diagnosis of an esophageal cause for the chest pain can be made on certain occasions. These are usually situations in which the patient demonstrates abnormal esophageal motility concurrent with pain or in which provocative testing (intraesophageal acid, edrophonium injection) reproduces the patient's symptoms. It is important to keep in mind that we too often fail in our ability to meet the challenge of providing definite diagnostic information in evaluating this group of patients. There are, however, some reasons for optimism in this area. With the newer technologies for measuring specific esophageal pressures, we are now better able to separate the normal from the abnormal esophageal contractions. In addition, there is presently an intense effort in a number of research laboratories to discover the more effective means of "stress testing" the esophagus to unmask motility abnormalities as a cause of these chest pain syndromes.

Exclude Diffuse Motility Disorder

As stated above, the esophageal motility abnormalities found in scleroderma are so specific and occur so commonly that one can often use motility testing to make a definite statement about the presence or absence of the disease. A similar situation applies to the patient with possible chronic idiopathic intestinal pseudo-obstruction. Definite abnormalities of esophageal motility have been demonstrated in a number of these patients.[21] They may present with a motility defect that may simulate achalasia, the abnormal esophageal motility that points to the specific diagnosis in a patient with a history of intermittent intestinal obstruction, or to its absence by providing strong evidence against this diagnosis.

Anorexia Nervosa

A recent publication has indicated that abnormal esophageal motility may be found in up to 50% of patients with a diagnosis of primary anorexia nervosa.[22] Many of these patients had previously undiagnosed achalasia. Following the manometric diagnosis, pneumatic dilatation resulted in weight gain. This observation strongly suggests that esophageal motility studies should be performed in all patients with a diagnosis of primary anorexia nervosa.

CONCLUSION

During the past decade, improvements in esophageal manometric techniques have provided the opportunity for more precise quantitative evaluation of esophageal motility. This has led to more specific identification of the manometric features of various esophageal motility abnormalities, and to improved diagnostic capability. The greater emphasis on investigative manometric studies has led to a widespread proliferation of clinical esophageal testing laboratories throughout this country. Two major phenomena have followed, and have had an important impact on the practicing physician. The first is a dramatic increase in the identification of patients with established or potential esophageal motility disorders. As esophageal laboratories have become more readily available, the referral of patients with dysphagia, chest pain, or heartburn has uncovered a great variety of potential esophageal motility abnormalities. In many patients, the manometric findings have resulted in confusion, often providing information of uncertain importance to the specific diagnosis or the cause of a patient's symptoms. The second major phenomenon arising from the proliferation of esophageal manometry laboratories is an increasing awareness of changing patterns of motility abnormalities in the same patient over a period of time. In this text we will attempt to provide insights into the proper application of today's manometric techniques and a brief overview of the clinical situations in which the esophageal manometry laboratory can be of value to the clinician.

REFERENCES

1. Kronecker H, Meltzer SJ: Der Schluckmechanismus, seine erregung and seine hummung. *Arch Ges Anat Physiol [Suppl]* 1883;7:328–332.
2. Meltzer SJ: Recent experimental contributions to the physiology of deglutition. *NY State J Med* 1894;59:389.
3. Ingelfinger FJ, Abbot WO: Intubation studies of human small intestine: Diagnostic significance of motor disturbances. *Am J Dig Dis* 1940;7:468–474.
4. Fyke FE, Code CF, Schlegel J: The gastroesophageal sphincter in healthy human beings. *Gastroenterologia (Basel)* 1956;86:135–150.
5. Pope CE: A dynamic test of sphincter strength: Its application to the lower esophageal sphincter. *Gastroenterology* 1967;52:779–786.
6. Winans CS, Harris LD: Quantitation of lower esophageal sphincter competence. *Gastroenterology* 1967;52:773–778.
7. Harris LD, Winans CS, Pope CE: Determination of yield pressures: A method for measuring anal sphincter competence. *Gastroenterology* 1966;50:754–760.
8. Cohen S, Harris LD: Lower esophageal sphincter pressure as an index of lower esophageal sphincter strength. *Gastroenterology* 1970;58:157–162.
9. Hollis JB, Castell DO: Amplitude of esophageal peristalsis as determined by rapid infusion. *Gastroenterology* 1972;63:417–422.

10. Stef JJ, Dodds WJ, Hogan WJ, et al: Intraluminal esophageal manometry: An analysis of variables affecting recording fidelity of peristaltic pressures. *Gastroenterology* 1974;67:221–230.
11. Arndorfer RC, Stef JJ, Dodds WJ, et al: Improved infusion system for intraluminal esophageal manometry. *Gastroenterology* 1977;73:23–27.
12. Waldeck F: A new procedure for functional analysis of the lower esophageal sphincter. *Pfluegers Arch* 1972;335:74–84.
13. Dodds WJ, Hogan WJ, Stef JJ, et al: A rapid pull-through technique for measuring lower esophageal sphincter pressure. *Gastroenterology* 1975;68:437–443.
14. Winans CS: Manometric asymmetry of the lower esophageal high pressure zone. *Am J Dig Dis* 1977;22:348–352.
15. Boyle JT, Altschuler SM, Nixon TE, et al: Role of the diaphragm in the genesis of lower esophageal sphincter pressure in the cat. *Gastroenterology* 1985;88:723–730.
16. Dent J: A new technique for continuous sphincter pressure measurement. *Gastroenterology* 1976;71:263–267.
17. Behar J, Biancani P, Sheahan DG: Evaluation of esophageal tests in the diagnosis of reflux esophagitis. *Gastroenterology* 1976;71:9–15.
18. Hollis JB, Castell DO: Effect of dry swallows and we swallows of different volumes on esophageal peristalsis. *J Appl Physiol* 1975;30:1161–1164.
19. Dodds WJ, Hogan WJ, Reid DP, et al: A comparison between primary esophageal peristalsis following wet and dry swallows. *J Appl Physiol* 1983;35:851–857.
20. Chobanian SJ, Castell DO: Esophageal abnormalities in systemic disease, in Castell DO, Johnson LF (eds): *Esophageal Function in Health and Disease.* New York, Elsevier Biomedical, 1983, pp 273–294.
21. Schuffler MD, Pope CE: Esophageal motor dysfunction in idiopathic intestinal pseudoobstruction. *Gastroenterology* 1976;70:677–682.
22. Stachner G, Kiss A, Wiesnagrotzki S, et al: Oesophageal and gastric motility disorders in patients categorized as having primary anorexia nervosa. *Gut* 1986;27:1120–1126.

CHAPTER **2**

Anatomy and Physiology of the Esophagus and Its Sphincters

Donald O. Castell, MD, FACP

ANATOMY

The human esophagus is a muscular tube whose major function is transport of food from the mouth to the stomach. It is bounded by a tonically contracted circular muscle sphincter at each end. The upper esophageal sphincter (UES) consists of striated muscle composed primarily of the cricopharyngeus muscle, but also aided by the inferior pharyngeal constrictors and the circular muscles of the upper esophagus. Because of the anterior attachments of the cricopharyngeus to the cricoid cartilage, the strongest contractile force in this sphincter is in the anterior-posterior direction, resulting in a slitlike configuration with the widest portion facing laterally.[1] The UES, like the striated musculature of the tongue, pharynx, and upper portion of the esophagus, is innervated like skeletal muscle, receiving motor input directly from the brain stem (nucleus ambiguus) to the motor endplates in the muscle (Fig. 2.1). The lower esophageal sphincter (LES) consists entirely of smooth muscle like most of the gastrointestinal (GI) tract. This sphincter is much more rounded in its closure, yet still demonstrates radial asymmetry, having higher pressures in the posterolateral direction.[2] Innervation of the LES is via efferent fibers that are carried through the vagus nerve and synapse in the myenteric plexus in the region of the LES.

The muscular wall of the esophagus is composed of an inner circular and an outer longitudinal layer. There is no serosa overlying the muscle layers. The UES and the upper portion of the tubular esophagus are primarily striated muscle. Recent studies have indicated that the transition from predominately striated to predominately smooth muscle occurs in the upper

13

4 to 5 cm of the human esophagus, although it is somewhat variable in different subjects and in the different muscle layers. Consistently, greater than the distal half of the human esophagus is entirely smooth muscle.[3] Like the LES, innervation of the smooth muscle portion of the tubular esophagus is primarily via the vagus nerve from neurons arising in the dorsal motor nucleus with nerve endings in the myenteric plexus (Fig. 2.1).

PHYSIOLOGY

Traditionally, swallowing or deglutition has been divided into three stages: the oral (voluntary) stage, the pharyngeal (involuntary) stage, and the esophageal stage. These three are, of course, closely coordinated and continuing processes that are regulated through the swallowing center in the medulla.[4]

Voluntary Stage

This is a process by which the swallowing mechanism is primed. Ingested food is voluntarily moved posteriorly by movements of the tongue muscles, forcing the food bolus towards the pharynx and pushing it backward and upward against the palate. Once the food has been delivered to the pharynx, the process becomes involuntary. This process obviously requires proper functioning of the striated muscles of the tongue and pharynx and is the stage of swallowing that is likely to be abnormal in patients with neurologic or skeletal muscle disease.

Pharyngeal Stage

During this stage of swallowing, the food is passed from the pharynx, across the UES, and into the proximal esophagus. This involuntary process requires the finely tuned coordinated sequences of contraction and relaxation, resulting in *transfer* of the ingested material. The presence of food in the pharynx stimulates sensory receptors, which send impulses to the swallowing center in the brainstem. The central nervous system (CNS) then initiates a series of involuntary responses that include the following:

1. The soft palate is pulled upward and *closes the posterior nares.*
2. The palatopharyngeal folds are pulled medially, limiting the opening through the pharynx. This will tend to restrict the passage of a larger bolus.
3. The vocal cords are closed and the epiglottis swings backwards and down to *close the larynx.*

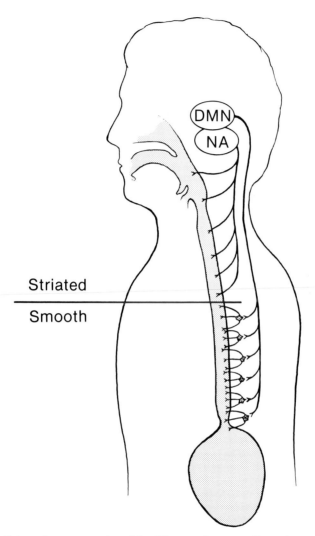

FIGURE 2.1 Schematic representation of the differences between efferent innervation of the striated muscle and smooth muscle portions of the human esophagus. Note that the striated muscle in the proximal esophagus receives direct input to motor endplates and that the cell bodies are located in the nucleus ambiguus (NA). In contrast, the smooth muscle portion, like that of the rest of the gastrointestinal tract, has indirect neural input into the muscles through the myenteric plexus. The ganglia originate in the dorsal motor nucleus (DMN) of the vagus nerve.

4. The larynx is pulled upward and forward by the muscles attached to the hyoid bone, stretching the opening of the esophagus and UES.
5. The *UES relaxes*. This is an *active relaxation* of the usually tonic cricopharyngeus combined with the passive opening created by the movement of the larynx.
6. Contraction of the superior constrictor muscle of the pharynx represents the beginning of the peristaltic wave that propels food into the esophagus.

This sequence is a coordinated mechanism that includes impulses carried by five cranial nerves. Sensory information to the swallowing center is carried along cranial nerves V, IX, and X. The motor responses from the swallowing center are carried along cranial nerves V, VII, IX, X, and XII. This intricate process takes approximately 1.5 sec from start to finish and requires coordination of pharyngeal contraction and UES relaxation (Fig. 2.2).

Esophageal Stage

The main function of the esophagus is to *transport* ingested material from the mouth to the stomach. This is an active process requiring contraction of both longitudinal and circular muscles of the tubular esophagus and coordinated relaxation of the sphincters. With the act of swallowing, the longitudinal muscle shortens during contraction to provide a structural base for the circular muscle contraction that forms the peristaltic wave. The sequential contraction of esophageal circular smooth muscle from proximal to distal generates the peristaltic clearing wave. The neuromuscular control of this activity will be described below. As opposed to other GI smooth muscle, the esophageal smooth muscle has a unique electrical activity pattern showing only spiked potentials without underlying slow waves. Circular muscle contractions can be characterized into three distinct patterns.

1. *Primary peristalsis.* This is the usual form of contraction wave of circular muscle that progresses down the esophagus and is initiated by the central mechanisms that follow the voluntary act of swallowing. It is a continuation of the wave that begins in the pharynx, and requires approximately 8 to 10 sec to reach the distal esophagus. These pressure relationships are shown in Figure 2.3.
2. *Secondary peristalsis.* This represents a peristaltic contraction of the circular esophageal muscle, which begins without central stimulation. This is to say, it originates in the esophagus as a result of distention and will usually continue until the esophagus is empty. Some food, particularly solid material, requires more than the single primary peristaltic wave for

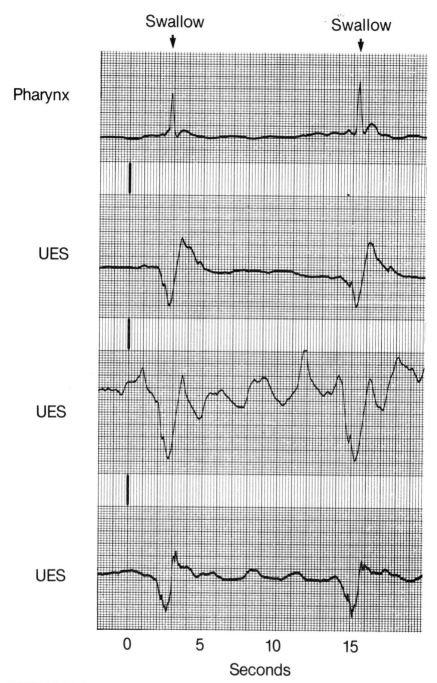

FIGURE 2.2 Motility tracing showing the coordinated sequence of contraction and relaxation between the human pharynx and UES. Here, the single opening recording pharyngeal pressure (top panel) is located 5 cm above the three lower openings located within the UES.

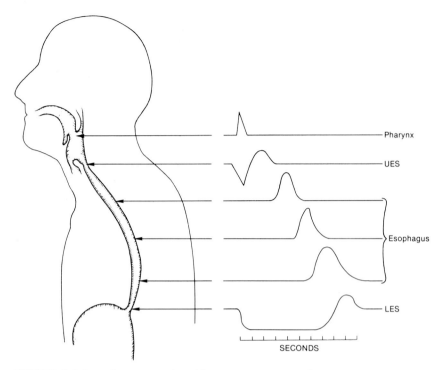

FIGURE 2.3 Schematic representation of the pressure sequence of a normal primary peristaltic wave. Note the single pressure complex that begins in the pharynx and progressively closes off the UES, then moves sequentially down the esophageal body and closes the LES. Also note that LES relaxation begins with the onset of the swallow and remains relaxed until the peristaltic wave reaches the distal esophagus (8 to 10 sec).

eventual clearance. This is accomplished by the secondary peristaltic waves. Thus, secondary peristalsis is the mechanism for clearing both ingested material and also material that is refluxed from the stomach. Experimentally, secondary peristalsis can be demonstrated by distending a balloon in the mid- to upper esophagus (Fig. 2.4).

3. *Tertiary contractions.* This contraction pattern is primarily identified during barium x-ray studies of the esophagus. It represents a nonperistaltic series of contraction waves that appear as localized segmented indentations in the barium column. It has no known physiologic function.

One of the interesting phenomena seen in the human esophagus occurs during the process of rapid sequential swallowing (usually less than 5 sec between successive voluntary swallows). This process results in inhibition of peristalsis, so-called "deglutitive inhibition." Peristalsis will be suspended during the continuation of a series of rapid swallows and a large "clearing wave" will occur at the completion of the swallows (Fig. 2.5). This phenomenon occurs because of the inhibitory neural discharge that arises from the central swallowing center during the voluntary act of swallowing, and also because the esophageal musculature shows a refractoriness, demonstrated to persist for up to 10 sec.[5]

Importance of the Esophageal Sphincters

The location of the esophagus in the thorax places it in a cavity that has negative pressure relative to the pharynx proximally and the stomach distally. The sphincters, therefore, must contain constant closure to prevent abnormal movement of air or food into the esophagus. In the absence of a tonically contracted UES, air will flow readily into the esophagus during inspiration. In the presence of a weak LES, gastric contents are not inhibited from refluxing readily into the distal esophagus, particularly in the recumbent position. Pressure relationships in and around the esophagus and its sphincters are shown in Figure 2.6.

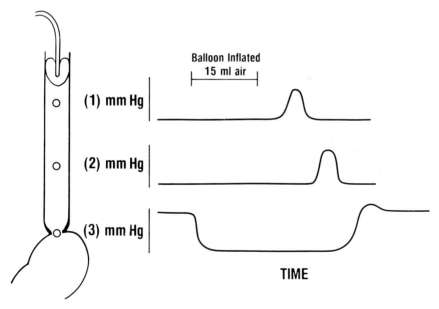

FIGURE 2.4 Demonstration of secondary peristalsis through the modality of inflation of a balloon in the proximal esophagus. During balloon inflation, the LES relaxes until a secondary peristaltic wave is produced at the time of deflation of the balloon.

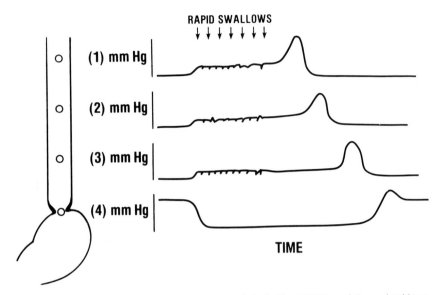

FIGURE 2.5 Demonstration of the phenomenon of deglutitive inhibition of the peristaltic sequence by rapid swallows separated by approximately 5-sec intervals. The LES remains relaxed throughout the sequence as the esophageal body is inhibited from a peristaltic response until the termination of the swallows. At this point the peristaltic clearing wave occurs.

Upper Esophageal Sphincter

The UES maintains a constant closure with strongest forces directed in the anterior-posterior orientation due to the attachment of the cricopharyngeus to the cricoid cartilage. Normal pressures in the UES are approximately 100 mm Hg in the anterior-posterior direction and approximately 50 mm Hg laterally.[1]

Lower Esophageal Sphincter

The tonically contracted region at the esophogastric junction normally maintains a closing pressure of 15 to 35 mm Hg greater than the intragastric pressure below. By convention, the LES pressure is measured as a gradient in mm Hg higher than intragastric pressure, which is used as a zero reference. At the time of swallowing, the LES relaxes promptly in response to the initial neural discharge from the swallowing center and stays relaxed until the peristaltic wave reaches the end of the esophagus and produces sphincter closure. During relaxation, the pressure measured within the sphincter falls approximately to the level of gastric pressure; this is by definition a "complete" relaxation. Although there has been much controversy over the years, it is now generally accepted that the LES does *not* have to be located within the diaphragmatic crus in order to maintain a constant closing pressure. Thus, the presence of a sliding hiatal hernia is not necessarily detrimental to the physiologic function of this sphincter.

The LES maintains two important physiologic functions; the first is its

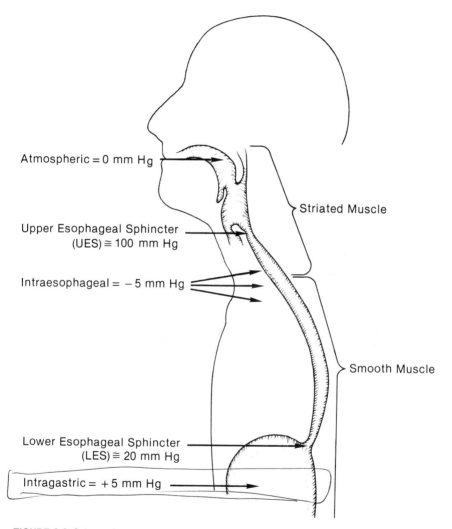

Atmospheric = 0 mm Hg

Striated Muscle

Upper Esophageal Sphincter (UES) ≅ 100 mm Hg

Intraesophageal = −5 mm Hg

Smooth Muscle

Lower Esophageal Sphincter (LES) ≅ 20 mm Hg

Intragastric = +5 mm Hg

FIGURE 2.6 Schematic representation of the pressure relationships in the pharynx, esophagus, esophageal sphincters, and stomach. Note the negative intraesophageal pressure relative to both pharyngeal (atmospheric) pressure and intragastric pressure. Thus, the importance of the sphincters in prevention of abnormal movement of fluids and air is emphasized.

role in prevention of gastroesophageal reflux and the second is its ability to relax with swallowing to allow movement of ingested material into the stomach. There has been considerable investigation and discussion regarding the mechanism by which the circular smooth muscle of the LES maintains tonic closure. At present, this is felt to be predominantly due to intrinsic muscle activity, since investigations in animals have identified that resting LES tone persists even after the destruction of all neural input by the neurotoxin tetrodotoxin.[6] In addition, truncal vagotomy does not affect resting LES pressure in humans. Calcium channel-blocking agents, which exert their effect directly on the circular smooth muscle, will produce decreases in LES pressures in animals and humans.[7,8] There also appears to be some cholinergic tone present in many animal species and in humans, since atropine will produce marked decreases in resting LES pressure.[9]

The mechanism of relaxation of the LES in response to a swallow has also been a subject of considerable investigation and controversy. The precise neurotransmitter responsible for this phenomenon is not definitely known. It is clear, however, that is not a classic cholinergic or adrenergic agent since specific pharmacologic blockade of these mechanisms does not inhibit LES relaxation. This is a neural event, however, since it can be reproduced in animals by stimulation of the vagus nerve and relaxation is inhibited by tetrodotoxin.[10] These relationships are summarized in Figure 2.7. There are recent studies suggesting that the neurotransmitter might be vasoactive intestinal polypeptide (VIP).[10]

It is important to understand the concept of a dynamic and frequently changing resting pressure in the LES. Pressures measured over long periods of time indicate that LES pressure will vary considerably, even from minute to minute. Much of this is due to the effect of a variety of factors that modulate pressure. These include foods ingested during meals and other events such as cigarette smoking and gastric distention (see Chapter 13). The normal LES will respond to transient increases in intra-abdominal pressure by raising its resting pressure to a greater degree than the pressure increases in the abdomen below. This is a protective mechanism intended to prevent gastroesophageal reflux. In addition, many hormones and other peptide substances produced in the GI tract and in other areas of the body have been shown to effect LES pressure. These are summarized in Table 2.1. It is important to recognize that many of these may represent primarily pharmacologic responses that have been shown to occur after intravenous injections or infusions of these substances in man or animals. Whether they represent truly physiologic actions has not been clarified in most cases. The strongest candidates for physiologic hormonal control of the LES are cholecystokinin, which explains the decreases in LES pressures seen after fat ingestion, and progesterone, which explains the decreases in LES pressure that may occur

LES RELAXATION

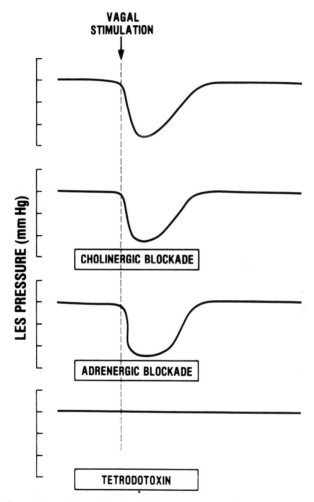

FIGURE 2.7 Summation of experiments in the opossum on the neural regulation of LES relaxation. Electrical stimulation of the vagus nerve produces relaxation, which is not inhibited by blocking either cholinergic or adrenergic pathways. The neural response is, however, inhibited by the neurotoxin tetrodotoxin.

TABLE 2.1 Effects of Peptides and Hormones on LES Pressure

Increases LES	Decreases LES
Gastrin	Secretin
Motilin	Cholecystokinin
Substance P	Glucagon
Pancreatic polypeptide	Gastric inhibitory
Bombesin	polypeptide (GIP)
Leu-enkephalin	VIP
Pitressin	Peptide histadine isoleucine
Angiotensin II	Progesterone

during pregnancy. Finally, there are various neurotransmitters and pharmacologic agents that have been shown to affect LES pressure. These are summarized in Table 2.2. Clearly, the modulation of LES resting pressure is a complex mechanism that involves the interaction of the LES smooth muscle, neural control, and humeral factors.[11]

Controls of Esophageal Peristalsis

As noted above, esophageal peristalsis is controlled via afferent and efferent neural connections through the swallowing center in the medulla. This central mechanism regulates the involuntary sequence of muscular events that occur during swallowing and simultaneously inhibits the respiratory center in the medulla so that respiration is stopped during all stages of swallowing.

The direct innervation to the striated muscle area of the pharynx and upper esophagus is carried via fibers from the brain stem (nucleus ambiguus) through the vagus nerve. The innervation to the smooth muscle of the distal esophagus and LES arises from the dorsal motor nucleus of the vagus and is carried through cholinergic visceral motor nerves to ganglia in the myenteric

TABLE 2.2 Effects of Neurotransmitters and Pharmacologic Agents on LES Pressure

Increases LES	Decreases LES
Cholinergic (bethanechol)	Dopamine
α-Adrenergic	β-Adrenergic
Metoclopramide	Atropine
	Nitrates
	Calcium-channel blockers
	Morphine
	Valium

plexis. There are also noncholinergic, nonadrenergic inhibitory nerves carried within the vagus.

The myenteric (Auerbach) plexus represents the esophageal portion of the enteric nervous system (the "brain in the gut"). The plexus receives efferent impulses from the central nervous system and sensory afferents from the esophagus. Thus, impulses travel in two directions through the myenteric plexus. This interconnecting and regulating way station is necessary for normal peristalsis in the smooth muscle esophagus. One manifestation of the afferent control is the observation that peristaltic squeezing pressures are regulated, to some degree, by the size of the ingested bolus. More important is the observation that dry swallows do not provide adequate stimulation for the production of true esophageal peristaltic pressures. The importance of the myenteric plexus as the primary regulatory mechanism of esophageal peristalsis in the smooth muscle portion is shown by observations that bilateral cervical vagotomy in animals does not abolish peristalsis in this area.

Interesting results have been obtained from in vitro studies of esophageal smooth-muscle preparations.[12] Using muscle from the opossum esophagus, it has been shown that the longitudinal smooth muscle demonstrates a sustained contraction during electrical field stimulation; this is called the "duration response." This response is neural and cholinergic since it can be blocked with both atropine and tetrodotoxin. The circular smooth muscle of the opossum esophagus shows a quite different response. With the onset of electrical stimulation there is a brief, small contraction at the beginning of the stimulus, known as the "on-response." This response is quite variable and has no known physiologic role. The on-response is followed by a much larger contraction that occurs after the termination of the stimulus, known as the "off-response." The off-response is also neural in origin, but is not cholinergic, since it is blocked only by tetrodotoxin and not atropine. Muscle strips taken from different segments of the smooth muscle portion of the esophageal body show progressively longer intervals for the off-response contraction following stimulation as one moves distally in the esophagus. This phenomenon has been called the "latency gradient." These concepts are shown in Figure 2.8.

It has been proposed that these in vitro experiments may help to explain some of the mechanisms of the development of normal peristalsis in the smooth-muscle esophagus. With the initial swallowing event, an inhibitory neural discharge is sent to the circular smooth muscle of the entire esophagus. The LES relaxes from its resting tonic state. The remainder of the esophageal smooth muscle is already relaxed and shows no measurable change. Rebound contraction occurs following the end of the brief stimulus (the off-response). The latency of the gradient for this off-response, progress-

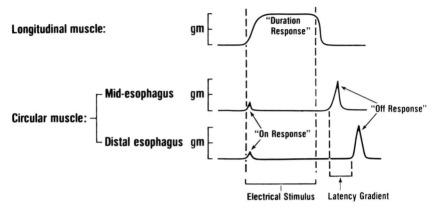

FIGURE 2.8 Summary of the in vitro esophageal smooth-muscle responses shown in experiments in the opossum. During stimulation the longitudinal esophageal muscle contracts throughout the stimulus; this is known as the duration response. The circular muscle shows a brief positive impulse at the beginning of stimulation; this is known as the on-response. This is followed by a much greater contraction following termination of the stimulus; this is known as the off-response. Delay in this latter response, progressing distally in the esophagus, produces the so-called latency gradient (gm = contraction force in grams).

ing distally down the esophagus, produces the peristaltic contraction wave. It is clear that this concept does not entirely explain all of the phenomena that have been observed in human peristaltic activity, but these in vitro observations are consistent with many aspects of normal human physiology. One example is the deglutitive inhibition referred to above. With repetitive swallowing at frequent intervals, the successive inhibitory neural impulses from the swallowing center prevent the contractions of the smooth-muscle portion of the esophagus until the last swallow occurs. The off-response and the latency gradient then allow the single peristaltic clearing wave that usually follows.

REFERENCES

1. Gerhardt DC, Shuck TJ, Bordeaux RA et al: Human upper esophageal sphincter. *Gastroenterology* 1978;75:268–274.
2. Winans CS: Manometric asymmetry of the lower esophageal high pressure zone. *Am J Dig Dis* 1977;22:348–354.
3. Meyer GW, Austin RM, Brady CE, et al: Muscle anatomy of the human esophagus. *J Clin Gastroenterol* 1986;8:131–137.
4. Weisbrodt NW: Neuromuscular organization of esophageal and pharyngeal motility. *Arch Intern Med* 1967;136:524–531.

5. Meyer GW, Gerhardt DC, Castell DO: Human esophageal response to rapid swallowing: muscle refractory period of neural inhibition? *Am J Physiol* 1981;241:G129–G136.
6. Goyal RK, Rattan S: Genesis of basal sphincter pressure: effect of tetrodotoxin on the lower esophageal sphincter in opposum in vivo. *Gastroenterology* 1976;71:62–67.
7. Richter JE, Sinar DR, Cordova CM et al: Verapamil–a potent inhibitor of esophageal function in baboons. *Gastroenterology* 1982;82:882–886.
8. Richter JE, Spurling TJ, Cordova CM, et al: Effects of oral calcium blocker, diltiazem, on esophageal contractions. *Dig Dis Sci* 1984;29:649–656.
9. Dodds WJ, Dent J, Hogan WJ, et al: Effect of atropine on esophageal motor function in humans. *Am J Physiol* 1981;240:G290–G296.
10. Goyal RK, Rattan S, Said SI: VIP as a possible neurotransmitter of non-cholinergic non-adrenergic inhibitory neurons. *Nature* 1980;288:370–380.
11. Castell DO: The lower esophageal sphincter: Physiologic and clinical aspects. *Ann Intern Med* 1975;83:390–401.
12. Christensen J, Lund GF: Esophageal responses to distention and electrical stimulation. *J Clin Invest* 1969;48:408–419.

CHAPTER **3**

The Esophageal Motility Laboratory
Materials and Equipment

Christine Boag Dalton, PA-C

The materials and equipment needed for an esophageal manometry lab can be divided into two general groups: the basic, or primary, equipment and the secondary equipment. The basic or primary equipment consists of a group of interconnected, relatively expensive, and essentially permanent pieces. The function of these pieces is to sense the activity of the muscles of the esophagus and to transmit and convert this to a permanent record that is easy to read and interpret. The basic equipment includes the esophageal manometry catheter, the infusion system, the transducers, and the physiograph. The secondary materials and equipment are relatively inexpensive and generally consumable items required to assist in the performance of the manometry study.

PRIMARY EQUIPMENT

The *esophageal manometry catheter* is a long flexible tube that is the only piece of equipment actually placed in the patient's esophagus. There are two main types: the water infusion type, in which the transducers are external, and the solid state type, in which the transducers are small and part of the catheter itself.

The *water-infusion system* consists of a catheter composed of several small capillary tubes. These tubes are continuously perfused with distilled water at a constant rate (0.5 mL/min) by a low-compliance pneumohydraulic capillary-infusion pump powered by compressed nitrogen. The individ-

28

ual capillary tubes are connected to external transducers that are, in turn, connected to the physiograph.

There are many different types of esophageal manometry catheters. The catheter used in our laboratory is described below and is recommended if our normal values are to be used as a standard. The catheter (available from Arndorfer Medical Specialties, Inc.) consists of eight capillary tubes (0.8-mm internal diameter) joined together around a larger central tube with a smooth outer surface (Fig. 3.1). The diameter of the entire catheter is 4.5 mm. Each of the eight capillary tubes has an opening or orifice at a set point along its length. These are the points where the pressure measurements are made. The eight orifices are numbered one through eight, with number one being the most distal (closest to the stomach while in use) and number eight the most proximal (closest to the mouth). The four distal orifices, numbers one through four, are 1 cm apart and oriented radially at 90° angles. Alternatively, we often use a tube with the four distal openings at the same level. Radial orientation helps to accurately measure lower esophageal sphincter (LES) pressures, which often have an assymmetrical pressure profile. These orifices are used primarily for LES determination. The four proximal orifices, numbers five through eight, are 5 cm apart and are also oriented at 90°

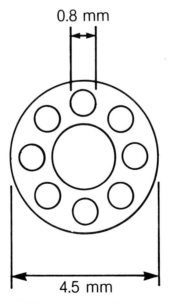

0.8 mm

4.5 mm

FIGURE 3.1 Cross-section of an 8-lumen esophageal manometry catheter showing the internal diameter of individual catheters and the diameter of the entire catheter.

angles (Fig. 3.2). These are used primarily for assessment of pressures in the body of the esophagus.

The other end of the catheter consists of the eight individual capillary tubes, each marked for identification and ending with a special tip for connection to the external transducers. The transducers are usually set on a rack at the same approximate level as the patient's esophagus in the supine position and are connected to both the infusion pump and the physiograph (Fig. 3.3). The infusion pump perfuses the catheters at a constant rate and pressure. When the individual catheter orifices are occluded (either by a contracting LES or a wave in the esophageal body), the pressure in the column of water changes and this is recorded by the external transducers. This pressure information is subsequently converted to an electrical signal by the transducer and printed out on the chart recorder.

The water infusion system is reliable and easy to use. The externally positioned transducers and infusion pump are easy to maintain and rarely break down. A broken transducer can be easily replaced and does not render the entire system inoperative. The patient must remain in the supine position with this system.

A *solid-state esophageal manometry catheter* usually has three microtransducers inside the catheter, which directly measure the pressure in the esophagus (Fig. 3.4). No water or infusion pump is used. The electrical signal from the transducers is carried by a cable attached to the physiograph. These catheters are routinely used by many labs, although we reserve their use for special situations. Since the microtransducers are positioned inside the patient's esophagus, studies may be performed in the upright or ambulatory positions. These catheters, however, do not offer the versatility of the water-perfused system because of the fixed placement of the transducers. Transducers break down frequently and are temperature sensitive. Malfunction of a single transducer requires that the entire system be sent for repair.

The *physiograph* receives the electrical signals from the transducers and the chart recorder produces the final printed tracing. The physiograph is usually the single most expensive piece of equipment. There are many types of physiographs and usually any system that works well can be used, if the following important criteria are met:

1. There should be at least four separate pressure-recording channels, since we use four ports of the catheter at all times. Having an extra channel for a swallow sensor and/or event marker is preferred.
2. Variable paper speeds are needed. The most useful are 1, 2.5, and 5 mm/sec.
3. Adjustable range for pressure measurement from a full scale of 50 to 100 mm Hg to a scale allowing at least 400 mm Hg.

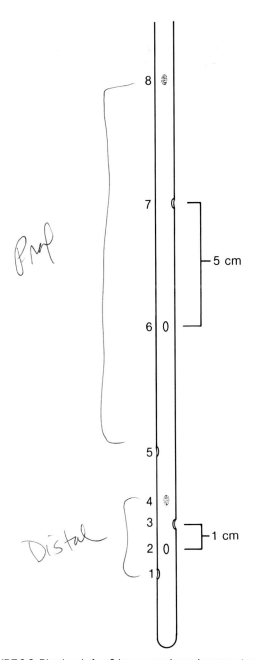

FIGURE 3.2 Distal end of an 8-lumen esophageal manometry catheter showing placement and orientation of all eight orifices.

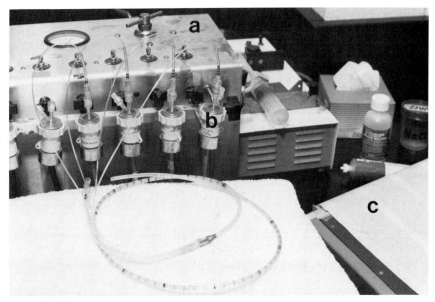

FIGURE 3.3 Primary equipment for esophageal manometry laboratory using the water-infusion system. Shown are (a) pneumohydraulic capillary-infusion pump, (b) external transducers, and (c) physiograph.

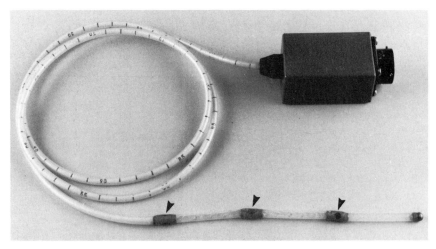

FIGURE 3.4 A solid-state esophageal manometry catheter with three microtransducers (arrows).

An event marker and a swallow signal are additional helpful accessories. We use a small microphone or electrodes taped to the neck to record swallows but a pneumograph belt in the form of a collar is also useful. We do not specifically record respirations, since they are evident on all pressure channels. Neither do we use a pH probe during the manometry study. Many companies have recently put together physiograph systems designed specifically for esophageal motility studies. Many offer accessories in addition to the basic equipment indicated above.

SECONDARY EQUIPMENT

The secondary equipment includes the materials and equipment, other than the previously discussed basic equipment, used during the esophageal motility testing. A mercury manometer is essential for accurate calibration of the transducers and physiograph. Viscous lidocaine, lubricating jelly, tissues, tape, an emesis basin (just in case), a 20-cc syringe or a straw with a container of room-temperature water, a penlight, and a tongue blade should be available for insertion of the tube (Fig. 3.5). We use the 20-cc syringe to give swallows of the water during the study. After the study, the tube, syringe, and water container are cleaned with a mild germicidal solution. Miscellaneous

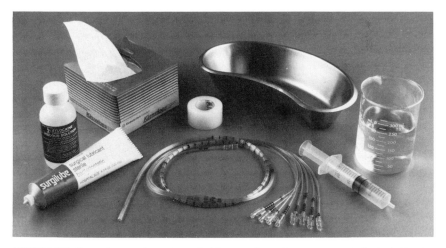

FIGURE 3.5 Secondary equipment needed for esophageal manometry study, including an 8-lumen esophageal manometry catheter.

equipment includes a stretcher or bed for the patient to lie on, a pillow, sheets, towels, and an intravenous (IV) pole.

Secondary materials used for special provocative testing include the following: (1) The Bernstein test requires three 60-cc syringes and 0.1N HCl and 0.9% saline solutions. A Harvard infusion pump can aide in the constant infusions of the solutions; (2) The edrophonium test requires 1-cc tuberculin syringes, alcohol swabs, edrophonium chloride, and atropine (the antidote to edrophonium).

CHAPTER **4**

The Manometric Study

Christine Boag Dalton, PA-C

It is important to remember that the esophageal manometry study is performed while the patient is awake and without sedation. Therefore everything must be done to insure the cooperation and comfort of the patient. This is essential for a successful study.

PREPARATION FOR THE STUDY

Before the first patient of the day arrives, it is important to calibrate the transducers and physiograph with a manometer that has a mercury column. Attach the manometer directly to a transducer with a three-way stopcock. Using a syringe full of air, apply varying amounts of pressure to the transducer while the physiograph is running (Fig. 4.1). Verify that the pressures recorded on the physiograph match the pressures shown on the manometer. Calibrate all transducers in this manner. This will ensure that your measurements are accurate.

The patient should fast for *at least* 4–6 hours before the study. Avoid doing the study on a patient who has eaten within the past four hours or has just had endoscopy (with sedation) or a barium upper gastrointestinal (GI) x-ray. The following medications should be discontinued 24 hours before the study, as they can interfere with normal esophageal function: nitrates (nitroglycerin, nitropatches, pastes, isosorbide dinitrate, etc), calcium channel-blocking agents (nifedipine, verapamil, diltiazem), anticholinergics (propantheline), promotility agents (metoclopromide, bethanechol), and sedatives (diazepam, etc). If the patient must continue a medicine that may

35

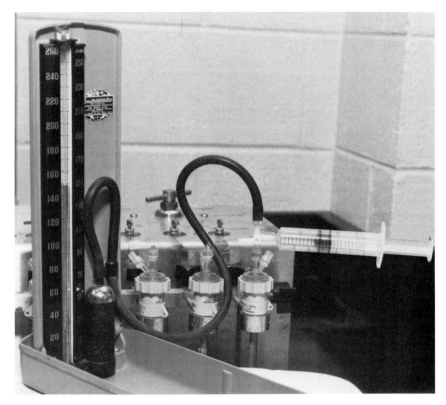

FIGURE 4.1 Calibration of the transducers and physiograph with a syringe full of air and a mercury manometer.

interfere with esophageal function, the study can still be done. However, make a note on the tracing and the final report explaining the situation.

At the beginning of the study, it is important to sit and talk with the patient for a few minutes. This helps to make the patient more comfortable and at ease about the procedure. We begin with a short history of the patient's chief complaint. We then ask about other esophageal and pulmonary symptoms, as well as prior esophageal and cardiac studies. *Always* take the time to explain to the patient what will happen during the study. A brief description is all that is needed and is very helpful in establishing patient rapport. Throughout this chapter, there will be extracted passages that are essentially *instructions to the patients*. These are not intended to be followed exactly, but are examples to use as guidelines and may be adapted for use in any laboratory.

I am going to do a study on your esophagus, or swallowing tube. I will take a small flexible tube, put it in one side of your nose, and gently move it back until it drops into the back of your throat. Then I will give you some water to swallow to help get the tube down. This can be uncomfortable, but once the tube is down, you will rapidly adjust to the feeling of the tube. I will give you time to get used to the tube before starting the actual study. The study begins with my moving the tube just a little to take some measurements. Then I will give you some swallows of water to see what your esophagus does when you swallow.

If doing the Bernstein test:

Next is a rest period where you swallow whenever you want.

If doing the edrophonium test:

Then there will be two injections of medicines that work on the type of muscles that make up the esophagus.

Finish your instructions with:

Finally, I will slowly pull the tube out while you swallow a few more times and we'll be through. It is important to tell me right away if, anytime during the study, you feel chest pain or heartburn.

Answer any questions the patient may have and prepare to put the tube down.

INTUBATION

This is probably the most uncomfortable part of the study for the patient. It is extremely important to do it gently and carefully. If you try to rush the intubation, you will get poor results and will spend even more time either waiting for the patient to settle down or trying to interpret a bad tracing.

Begin by having the patient remove glasses and any plates or dentures. Next, ask if they have a preference as to which side of the nose should be used. *A note here about nose versus mouth intubation:* To most people, the thought of a tube into the nose seems quite unpleasant and they think they would rather have the tube go through the mouth. The nasal route might be a little more uncomfortable during insertion, but it is *much* more tolerable for the remainder of the study. In nasal insertion, the tube hangs down the posterior pharynx, out of the way of the tongue and teeth. In oral insertion, the tube lies over the teeth and across the back of the tongue, causing constant mild discomfort and a greater tendency for the patient to gag.

Lubricate the tube immediately prior to insertion. We use 2% viscous lidocaine at the tip (ask if the patient is allergic) and regular lubricating jelly on the rest of the tube to about the 50-cm mark. Next, gently place the tip of the catheter into the nose and slowly move it *straight back*. Remember that the floor of the nose is flat (Fig. 4.2) and if you go *up* the nose you will cause

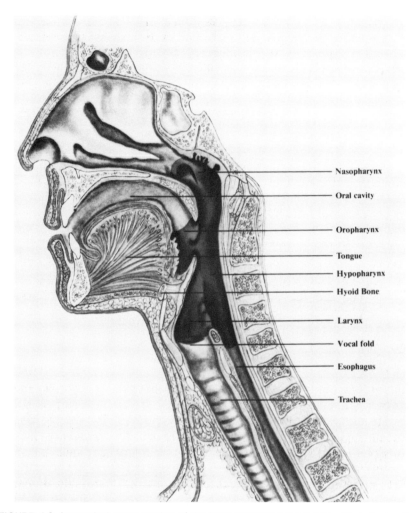

Nasopharynx

Oral cavity

Oropharynx

Tongue

Hypopharynx

Hyoid Bone

Larynx

Vocal fold

Esophagus

Trachea

FIGURE 4.2 Anatomical cross-section of the head illustrating the relationship between the pharynx and esophagus and demonstrating that the floor of the nose is flat.

your patient discomfort and get nowhere. When you get to the back of the nose, have the patient bend his neck down (chin to chest) to help the tube drop into the back of the throat. At this point, pay close attention to how your patient is acting. If he seems very uncomfortable or anxious, hold the tube in place for a few moments while you instruct the patient to take a few slow deep breaths. This should help relieve his anxiety. When the tip of the tube is in the back of the throat, give the patient some water to drink with a straw or syringe. As the patient swallows, rapidly advance the tube into the esophagus. It should easily enter the esophagus and *not* be associated with a lot of coughing (this symptom suggests intubation of the trachea). If you do not get into the esophagus, pull back and let the patient catch his breath before repeating the intubation attempt. When the tube first enters the esophagus, it may be uncomfortable for the patient. Having him take a few deep breaths will decrease the discomfort. As you continue to advance the tube, reassure the patient:

You are doing fine . . . take a deep breath . . . the worst is over.

When the 50-cm mark on the tube is at the tip of the nose, the end of the tube will be either in the stomach or just above the lower esophageal sphincter (LES). If you are unable to pass the catheter through the LES and into the stomach, continue the attempt while twisting the tube slightly. Then try giving swallows of water to the patient or have the patient take a deep breath. If the patient has a history of trouble swallowing he may use a special maneuver that often helps to pass the catheter. Tape the tube to the nose, trying to keep the tube away from the nasal septum. Help the patient lie down and tell him to relax and use the next 5 to 10 minutes to get accustomed to the tube. Connect catheter tips one through four to the transducers and turn on the water at the infusion pump.

THE MANOMETRIC STUDY

Double check your equipment (knobs, dials, gauges, water level, etc) before beginning the study to make sure that everything is on the right setting and is ready to begin. Label the tracing with the patient's name and hospital number and the date. As the study progresses, it is very important to make a note on the tracing every time something is done, eg, change of scale, moving tube to new position, cough, wet swallow, etc. This will make it much easier to interpret the tracing at a later time.

To begin the study, first verify that all perfused ports are in the stomach. To do this, turn on the physiograph at a paper speed of 2.5 mm/sec. You should see something similar to Figure 4.3 in *all four* channels; a relatively flat smooth tracing with a small pressure increase moving upward on inspiration. This confirms placement in the stomach and is referred to as the gastric baseline. Ask the patient to take in a deep breath while you watch the tracing. If the tracing goes *down* with inspiration, the ports are in the esophagus, not the stomach. If portions of the tracing go up while others go down, or if all go up but not all are smooth and flat, then the catheter is partially in the sphincter and you need to advance the tube further down. Once again, make sure the patient is feeling fairly comfortable with the tube before beginning the study. If not, a few more minutes of waiting should help.

One or more of the channels may be unresponsive and show a straight line (Fig. 4.4). This can be caused by several factors. First, check that the

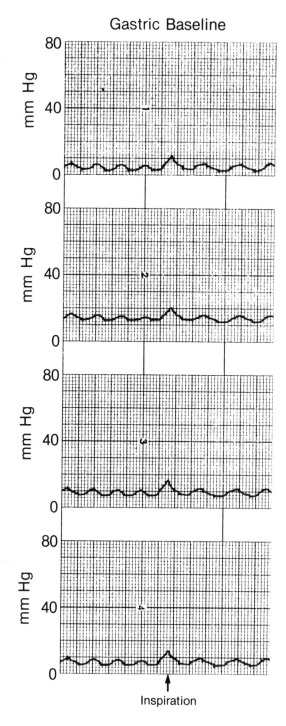

FIGURE 4.3 Motility recording with four openings in the stomach showing quiet respiration and a *rise* in pressure during inspiration.

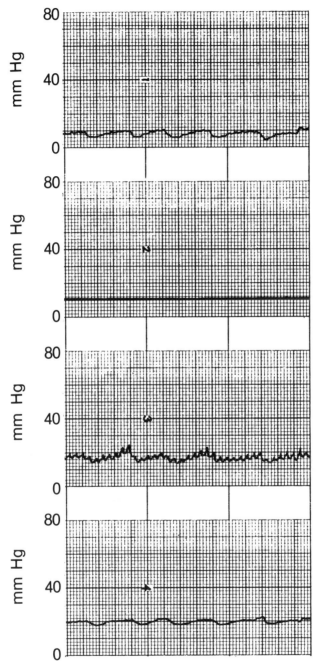

FIGURE 4.4 Motility recording showing a straight line in one channel, indicating an unresponsive lead.

water from the infusion pump is on and flowing. Next, insure that the catheter orifice is not blocked by injecting water through the tip. The catheter may be curled or bent, especially if you had a lot of trouble getting it down. Encountering a great deal of resistance when you move the tube indicates that this may be the problem. Advance the tip further into the stomach. If the tip is curled, it will have the room to straighten out inside the stomach. If this does not help and you feel certain the equipment is not malfunctioning, you may have to totally remove the catheter and start over.

THE LOWER ESOPHAGEAL SPHINCTER

Remember that the smooth muscle of the LES is normally contracted to maintain closure, and that the LES opens or relaxes with a swallow. We measure the LES with both the rapid pull-through (RPT) and the station pull-through (SPT) techniques.

   The RPT technique measures LES pressure as the catheter is pulled from the stomach, across the LES, and into the esophagus. This is done while the patient is not breathing or swallowing. Before beginning let the patient know what to expect:

> I am going to slowly pull the tube out a few inches. While I am pulling the tube, I do not want you to breathe or swallow. Before beginning, I will tell you to take a breath, let it out, and hold it. You do not need to take a deep breath or to hold your breath hard. You will only be asked to hold your breath for about 10 – 15 seconds.

   While holding the catheter close to the patient's nose, start the physiograph at 2.5 mm/sec. Tell the patient to take a breath, let it out, and hold it. Slowly pull the tube out (1 – 2 cm/sec) while watching the tracing. You should see a rise in pressure (the LES) and then a drop in pressure to *below* the gastric baseline as you enter the esophagus. (Note: esophageal pressure is lower than gastric pressure because of the relatively negative pressures within the chest cavity.) At this point, *stop* pulling the tube and tell the patient to take a breath. The tracing should look similar to Figure 4.5. Read the distance on the tube and make a note on the tracing. Gently move the tube back into the stomach, wait 1 – 2 min, and repeat the RPT. Because this can be uncomfortable for the patient, we usually only perform two RPTs. If they look very different, a third may be needed. The final LES pressure is the mean value of the eight individual pressures from two similar pull-throughs. There are several things that can "throw off" an RPT (see Chapter 5). The advantages of the RPT technique are that it is easy and fast, identifies the location of the LES, gives you a general feel for the pressures in the sphincter, and can be performed in the patient who swallows frequently.

The SPT technique gives a more complete assessment of LES function. With this technique, the catheter is moved through the LES 0.5 cm at a time, with a pause at each point or station, to closely observe LES pressure and relaxation. If you had trouble passing the catheter into the stomach or have a patient with possible achalasia (a disorder with a poorly relaxing LES), *begin* the study with the SPT, in case you are unable to enter the stomach a second time. Before beginning, tell the patient what you will be doing:

> I'm going to slowly pull the tube out a little at a time. I want you to just relax and concentrate on breathing *regularly* and *evenly*. Try to swallow as little as possible.

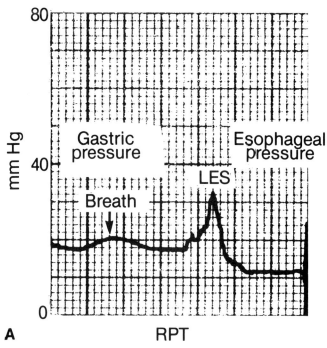

FIGURE 4.5 (A) RPT of the LES. This figure shows the detailed tracing obtained from one orifice during one breath and then during breath-holding, as the opening of the catheter is pulled from the stomach, through the LES, and into the esophagus. Note that esophageal pressure is lower than gastric pressure. Figure 4.5B continued on p. 44.

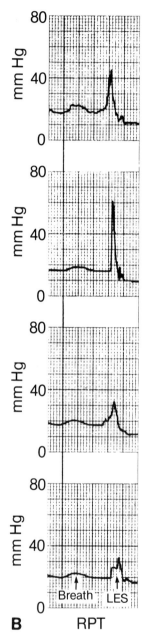

FIGURE 4.5 (B) RPT of the LES showing the results of recording from four orifices. This illustration clearly shows the radial asymmetry of the LES.

As before, begin with all ports in the stomach. Hold the catheter close to the nose and steady your hand on the patient's chin. This gives you good control of the catheter and is more comfortable for the patient. If the patient is still swallowing frequently, you might want to wait a few more minutes before beginning. Start the physiograph at a paper speed of 1 mm/sec and record on the tracing the location of the tube. Move the tube out 1 cm, record the distance, and examine the tracing. If the tracing is unchanged, move the tube another centimeter. Continue to do this until you see an increase in the baseline pressure on the tracing, which corresponds with the patient's breathing. This exaggerated respiratory variation is seen while the port is in the LES (Fig. 4.6) because of the close proximity of the sphincter to the diaphragm. Now begin to move the catheter 0.5 cm at a time. Remain at each position or station, for at least 3–5 respiration cycles, noting the activity in all four leads. As you move further into the LES, the bottom of the pressure complex will usually rise above the gastric baseline. At this point, an assessment of sphincter relaxation can be made. As you ask the patient to swallow,

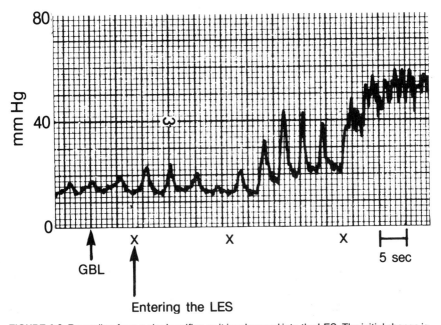

FIGURE 4.6 Recording from a single orifice as it is advanced into the LES. The initial change is an exaggeration of the respiratory variations from the gastric baseline (GBL), with subsequent elevation of the entire pressure profile as the catheter is moved upward. x, tube moved up 0.5 cm.

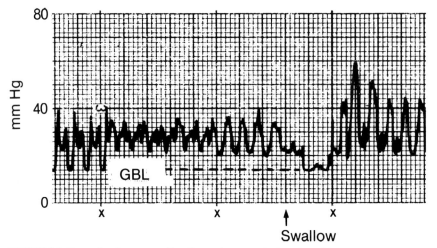

FIGURE 4.7 Recording from one orifice illustrating normal relaxation of the LES during an SPT. Note that the pressure falls to the level of the GBL for a period of greater than 5 sec. Paper speed is 1 mm/sec. x, tube moved up 0.5 cm.

watch for a drop in pressure to *about* the level of the gastric baseline (Fig. 4.7). If relaxation does not appear complete (does not go down to gastric baseline) give the patient a 5-cc swallow of water. The *normal* lower sphincter should always relax completely to gastric pressure with a wet swallow. Even if the respiratory variations are not off the baseline, you will

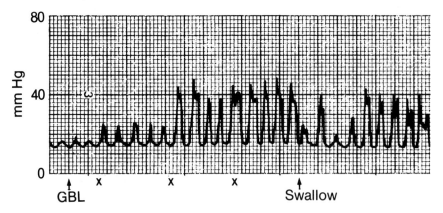

FIGURE 4.8 Recording from single orifice demonstrating LES sphincter relaxation during swallowing on an SPT in a patient with a low sphincter pressure. Although a clear drop in pressure cannot be identified in this patient, since the sphincter pressure has not risen completely above the gastric baseline, there is a clear change in the wave pattern following the swallow. x, tube moved up 0.5 cm.

see a change in the waveform with a swallow (Fig. 4.8). Following a swallow during the SPT, spend more time (8–10 sec) at that station to allow the effects of the swallow to clear.

As you continue through the LES, stopping at 0.5-cm intervals, you will soon come to a point where the tracing goes *down rather than up with inspiration.* This is the *pressure inversion point* (PIP), also known as the *point of respiratory reversal* (Fig. 4.9). This occurs as the port moves from the abdominal cavity into the thoracic cavity. If you are measuring a very weak or low-pressure sphincter, this reversal point may be the only way to locate

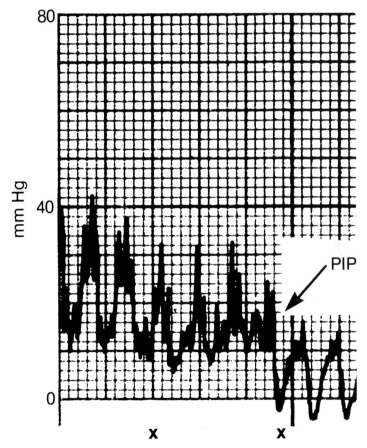

FIGURE 4.9 Recording from a single orifice of LES pressure during an SPT, demonstrating PIP. The pressure deflection has changed dramatically from upward to downward with inspiration. x, tube moved up 0.5 cm.

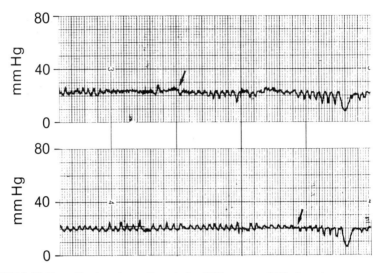

FIGURE 4.10 Recording from two orifices during SPT across an LES of very low pressure. The location of the sphincter is only clearly identified by the distinct PIP shown at the arrows. Paper speed is 1 mm/sec.

the LES (Fig. 4.10). The PIP is occasionally preceded by a period when the tracing moves *both up and down* with inspiration (Fig. 4.11). It is important to remember that you are still in the LES, even though the tracing is in reversal. Once the pressure tracing is in reversal, you have probably passed the highest LES pressure and will find that the pressure will continue to drop as you move out of the LES and into the esophagus. When the most distal of the four ports has entered the body of the esophagus (Fig. 4.12), note the measurement where the stable baseline begins, adjust the catheter to 3 cm above that point, and tape the tube in place. Change the connections from ports 1, 2, 3, 4 to ports 1, 5, 6, 7 and label the tracing. You are now ready to assess the body of the esophagus.

THE BODY OF THE ESOPHAGUS

The study of the body of the esophagus evaluates the muscle response to a swallow. Normally, the muscles contract in an orderly sequence from top to bottom (peristalsis) in order to push the swallowed bolus into the stomach. For this portion of the study, the perfused ports are 5 cm apart, with the most

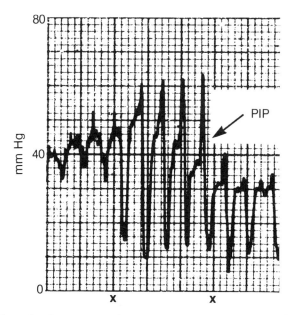

FIGURE 4.11 Recording from a single orifice showing variation in PIP. A biphasic change will often be seen. This is intermediate between the upward deflection with respiration, representing intra-abdominal pressure (left), and the downward deflection with respiration, representing intrathoracic pressure (right). X, tube moved up 0.5 cm.

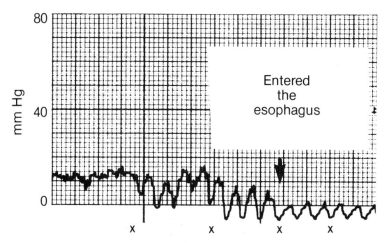

FIGURE 4.12 Recording from a single orifice demonstrating the transition in pressures across the PIP into the esophagus during an SPT. As the orifice leaves the lower esophageal sphincter and enters the body of the esophagus, the tracing shows a drop in pressure and then a stable pressure that does not change with continued upward movement of the catheter. x, tube moved up 0.5 cm.

distal (1) being 3 cm above the LES. This will leave ports 5, 6, and 7 at 8 cm, 13 cm, and 18 cm above the LES, respectively (Fig. 4.13). While you are waiting for the tubes to perfuse, tell the patient what will happen next:

> For the next part of the study, you will be given swallows of water, about a teaspoon at a time. Collect the water in the back of your throat and swallow just one time to get it down. I will be giving you swallows every 30 seconds. Try to keep from swallowing on your own.

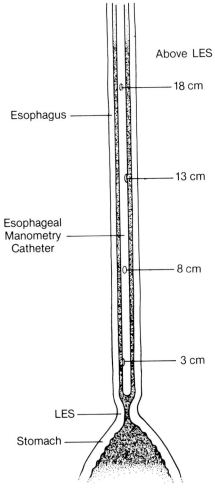

FIGURE 4.13 Schematic representation illustrating the placement of the recording catheter for assessment of esophageal body pressures. Recording orifices are located 3, 8, 13, and 18 cm above the LES.

Turn the physiograph on, at a paper speed of 2.5 mm/sec. Using a syringe and room-temperature water, place a 5-cc bolus of water in the patient's mouth and ask him to swallow once. Watch the tracing to see the response of the esophagus to the swallow. You may need to increase the pressure range on the physiograph, if the contraction flattens out instead of coming to a peak. Check the proximal (top) lead and turn it off if it is in the upper esophageal sphincter (UES) (Fig. 4.14). If the patient has not swallowed

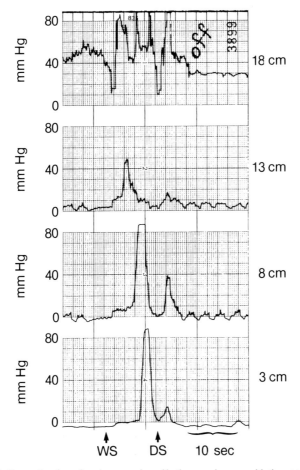

FIGURE 4.14 Recording from four lumens placed in the esophagus, with the proximal orifice at the UES. This tracing illustrates the relaxation of the upper sphincter during both a wet (WS) and dry (DS) swallow. The water infusion to the proximal orifice is turned off to decrease patient discomfort. The tracing also demonstrates the higher pressures recorded in the more distal esophagus (channels labeled 3 cm and 8 cm), which necessitate an increase in the range setting.

spontaneously after 30 sec, give another 5-cc water bolus. A normal tracing of a swallow should resemble Figure 4.15., with an orderly progression of contractions from top to bottom known as *peristalsis*. It takes most patients a few practice swallows to get used to this procedure, so we routinely give a total of 15 swallows and interpret only the last ten swallows. Do not forget to label all wet swallows, dry swallows, and anything else that affects the tracing. Give at least 15 swallows, and more if there might be a question later.

If the patient appears to be having difficulty with the water, you may

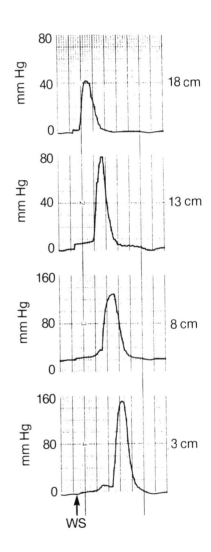

FIGURE 4.15 Recording with four orifices placed in the body of the esophagus illustrating a normal peristaltic sequence in response to a wet swallow (WS).

give as little as 3 cc. If the patient continues to dry swallow before the next wet swallow, you may give the water as frequently as every 20 sec.

If the contractions appear to happen at the same time (simultaneous) or from the bottom to top (retrograde), first *check the catheter connections* to the transducer to verify that the correct changes were made. If the connections are correct, the patient may have an esophageal motility disorder. If the contractions appear simultaneous, increase the paper speed to 5 mm/sec and continue to give wet swallows. This will "spread out" the tracing of the contraction and will make it easier to determine if the contractions are simultaneous or peristaltic (Fig. 4.16). If the tracing appears to show repeti-

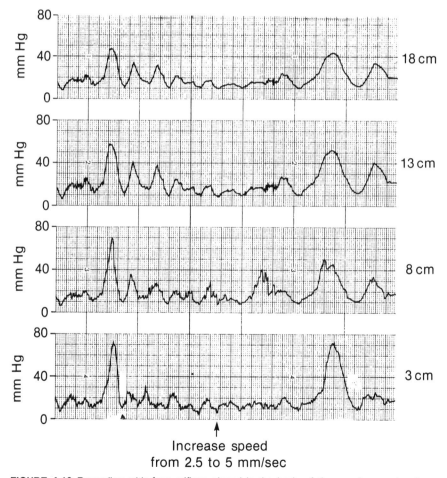

FIGURE 4.16 Recording with four orifices placed in the body of the esophagus showing possible simultaneous contractions, which are more readily identified by increasing the paper speed.

tive (multi-peaked) contractions, these may only be respirations. Ask the patient to hold his breath as soon as you see repetitive activity. If the activity continues, it is not a result of respiratory movement (Fig. 4.17).

If the patient coughs during the study, stop what you are doing and ask that he cough as much as needed to get comfortable again. You do not want the patient to be suppressing a cough while you are doing the study.

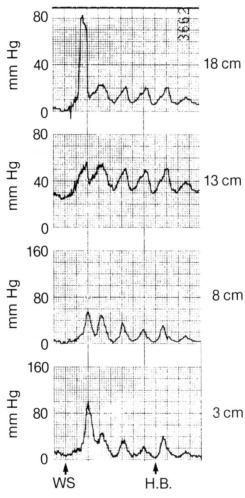

FIGURE 4.17 Recording with four orifices placed in the body of the esophagus. Example of the repetitive simultaneous contractions of low amplitude resembling respiratory variations. The pressure deflections continue with the patient holding his/her breath (H.B.). WS, wet swallow.

You may see very rapid activity in one or more of the channels (Fig. 4.18). This interference is often caused by the heart. It is frequently seen in the orifice at 13 cm above the LES, which may be adjacent to the aortic arch. Interference more rapid than the heart rate may be electrical or 60-cycle activity. Readjusting the catheter position by a small amount or increasing the range may minimize or eliminate the activity on the tracing.

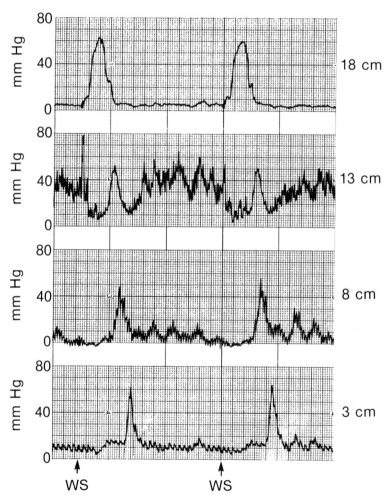

FIGURE 4.18 Recording with four orifices placed in the body of the esophagus demonstrating cardiac interference at the site located 13 cm and, to a lesser degree, 8 cm above the LES. During the two wet swallows (WS) the peristaltic wave is still clearly identified in this area.

PROVOCATIVE TESTING

Provocative testing is an optional part of the esophageal manometry study. It is used to bring out or reproduce symptoms that might be esophageal in origin. Interpretation is based on the patient's subjective complaints rather than a specific manometric change. Because of this subjective factor, the provocative tests must have a blinded placebo phase. It is important not to draw any special attention to this part of the test. Inform the patient at the beginning of the manometric study that he should tell you if he experiences any symptoms, and periodically remind him of this throughout the study.

The *Bernstein test* is used to assess the acid sensitivity of the esophagus. It is done by perfusing acid and/or saline directly through the catheter into the esophagus. We tell the patient that this is a rest period and they can swallow as needed. Label your tracing and slow the paper speed to 0.25 mm/sec in order to save paper. Begin by infusing normal saline through the No. 3 port (5 cm above the LES) at a rate of 7–8 cc/min for a few minutes. Next infuse 0.1N HCl through the same port at the same rate. If you give all 80 cc of acid over 10 min without a complaint of heartburn or chest pain from the patient, you have a *negative* Bernstein test. If the patient complains of heartburn or chest pain, quietly switch back to saline. A *true-positive test* requires that the symptoms ease or leave with the saline infusion and return or worsen with a second acid infusion. Anything in between is just described on the report form and called *equivocal*.

The *edrophonium test* consists of two injections: 0.9% normal saline (the placebo) and edrophonium chloride, a short-acting cholinesterase inhibitor that increases the amplitude and duration of esophageal contractions. We tell the patient that he will receive two injections, with each followed by more swallows of water. We describe the injections as medicines that work specifically on the muscles of the esophagus. We remind him again to report any symptoms he may feel.

Begin with an injection of 0.2 cc of 0.9% NaCl, either IV or SQ. Follow this with four swallows of water, as before. Record the symptoms. The amount of edrophonium to be given is determined by the patient's weight and the following formula:

$$\frac{\text{Patient weight}}{2.2} \times 0.008 = \text{Number of cc of edrophonium}$$

For example, if the patient weighs 150 lb,

$$\frac{150 \text{ lb}}{2.2} = 68 \text{ kg}$$

$$68 \times 0.008 = 0.54 \text{ cc}$$

This is based on giving a 10 mg/mL solution. Therefore, the number of cubic centimeters times 10 equals the number of milligrams of (0.54 cc = 5.4 mg). We do not use more than 1.0 cc of edrophonium, even if the patient's weight warrants it.

The injection of edrophonium *must* be intravenous. If the patient complains of burning at the injection site, the drug is not going into the vein. Following the injection, give the patient ten swallows of water at 30-sec intervals. A positive test occurs when the patient complains of his typical chest pain after the injection. Many times there will be an association between the patient's complaint of pain and the presence of a high-amplitude long-duration contraction in the esophagus. The chest pain is usually mild in intensity.

Some patients may complain of side effects from the edrophonium. The most common effects include watery eyes, dizziness, and abdominal cramping. Reassure the patient that the discomfort will pass quickly. We *do not* give edrophonium to patients with a recent history of asthma, chronic obstructive lung disease, or cardiac arrhythmia. The antidote to edrophonium is atropine. We keep a syringe with 1-mg atropine sulfate close at hand, although we have never needed to use it.

UPPER ESOPHAGEAL SPHINCTER

The assessment of the UES is the final part of the esophageal manometry study and is done during withdrawal of the catheter. The UES, like the LES, has a high resting pressure and relaxes with a swallow. However, the UES is composed of striated muscle and the LES is composed of smooth muscle. Because of this difference, the relaxation phase of the UES is much more rapid, necessitating a faster paper speed. When you are ready to begin withdrawing the catheter, turn the paper speed to 5 mm/sec and the range to around 100 mm Hg. Slowly pull the catheter out while watching the proximal baseline. When you see a rise in pressure, stop and watch the tracing for a few seconds before asking the patient to swallow. The normal response to a swallow is a U-shaped drop in pressure to the esophageal baseline, followed by a rise in pressure higher than the original pressure, and a return to UES pressure (Fig. 4.19). We usually give two swallows at each level and then pull forward until the next port is in the UES. At this point, the proximal port is in the pharynx. Now with a swallow you can assess not only relaxation of the UES, but also its coordination with the pharyngeal contraction. The peak of the pharyngeal contraction occurs during the trough of the UES relaxation (Fig. 4.20). It is important to remember that this is a qualitative assessment.

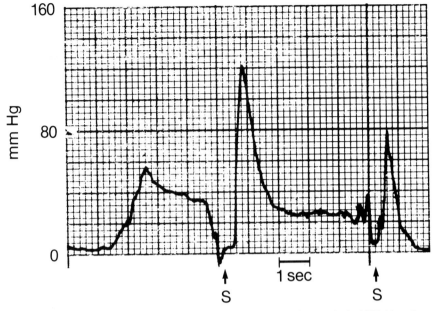

FIGURE 4.19 Recording from a single orifice showing pressure changes in the UES. Note that with each swallow (S) there is a rapid decrease in pressure followed by a subsequent increase (the "post swallowing augmentation"). Paper speed is 5 mm/sec.

We do not routinely measure UES pressures (see Chapter 14) and it is not possible to accurately measure the pharyngeal contraction with a perfused catheter. Continue to assess the UES with each port as you withdraw the catheter. Remember to turn off the water to each port as it clears the pharynx, since the fluid will accumulate in the back of the throat and cause the patient to cough.

After the tube is completely withdrawn from the patient, disconnect it from the infusion pump. Tell the patient to relax and catch his breath as you quickly rinse off the catheter and inject water through the individual capillary tubes. It is important to do this immediately following the study to prevent any clogging of the ports by dried secretions. Final washing of both the inside and outside of the catheter with a mild germicidal solution (do not soak the tube), followed by a thorough rinsing and drying, leaves the tube ready for the next study.

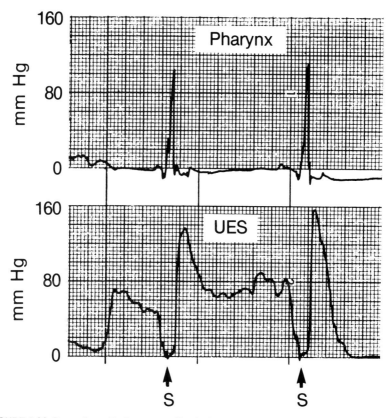

FIGURE 4.20 Recording with the upper orifice in the pharynx 5 cm above the lower orifice in the UES. Note the rapid sequence of UES relaxation and pharyngeal contraction with each swallow (S). Paper speed is 5 mm/sec.

You may want to discuss the results of the test with the patient. Patients usually enjoy seeing the tracing and receiving a brief explanation of what it shows.

A condensed version of the technique for a complete esophageal manometry study is shown in Table 4.1 (see p. 60).

Table 4.1 Esophageal Manometry Technique

Lower esophageal sphincter (LES) pressure[a]
  RPT
    Do two
    End expiration
    Pull rate: 1–2 cm/sec
    Paper speed: 2.5 mm/sec
    Mean of 8 values
  SPT
    0.5-cm increments 3–5 respirations/station
    Assess relaxation with dry swallows and add wet swallows if in doubt about relaxation
    Paper speed: 1 mm/sec
    Mean of 4 values

Esophageal body[b]
  Recording sites 3, 8, 13, and 18 cm above LES
  15 wet swallows (5 cc H_2O) at 30-sec intervals
  Calculate amplitude and duration as mean of last 10 swallows
  Paper speed: 2.5 mm/sec

Provocative testing
  Bernstein test (used to assess acid sensitivity)
    Patient supine with perfusion port (use port 3) 5 cm above LES
    Infusion rate 7–8 mL/min; swallows as needed
    NaCl for 2 to 3 min
    0.1N HCl for 10 min (80 mL)
    Record symptoms, if any, and infuse NaCl until symptoms ease, then repeat HCl to
      reproduce symptoms for true-positive test
  Edrophonium chloride test (a drug that increases the amplitude and duration of
      contractions of the esophagus)
    NaCl injection of 0.2 cc; give 4 wet swallows and record symptoms
    Tensilon injection of 80 μg/kg IV, followed immediately by 10 wet swallows
    Record symptoms and try to correlate symptoms with contractions
    Formula: (Patient wt in lb ÷ 2.2) × (0.008) = # of cc needed
    Antidote: atropine

UES
  Primarily to assess coordination/relaxation
  Paper speed: 5–10 mm/sec

[a]Use ports 1, 2, 3, and 4.
[b]Use ports 1, 5, 6, and 7.

CHAPTER 5

Measurements and Interpretations

Christine Boag Dalton, PA-C

Careful and accurate measurement of esophageal manometry tracing is essential for a correct interpretation and diagnosis of esophageal motility disorders. Although the measurements themselves are not difficult, each part of the test is done differently and this at first might be confusing. The actual measurements are usually made after the completion of the study. It is important to remember that the tracing should be well marked, from beginning to end, and should include information regarding all changes of scale, paper speed, and complaints of pain or burning from the patient. Accurate and copious notations on the tracing insure fewer questions.

LOWER ESOPHAGEAL SPHINCTER PRESSURE

Measurements are made in millimeters of mercury (mm Hg), using gastric baseline (GBL) as the reference point (0 mm Hg). The rapid pull-through (RPT) technique measures lower esophageal sphincter (LES) pressure during suspended respiration from GBL to the peak of the pressure rise (Fig. 5.1). We perform two RPTs, providing four pressure readings from each. The average of the eight values represents the mean LES pressure (Fig. 5.2).

As mentioned in Chapter 4, the RPT measurements can be easily thrown off and an abnormally high or low pressure can result. If the tube is pulled too rapidly or the patient bears down, which can happen if the tube is pulled too slowly, an abnormally high RPT pressure can result. An abnor-

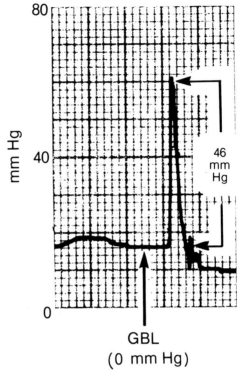

FIGURE 5.1 Rapid pull-through technique measures LES pressure during suspended respiration from GBL (0 mm Hg) to the peak of pressure rise. The numbers to the left represent the range setting on the physiograph.

mally low RPT pressure can result if the patient swallows before the pull-through.

LES pressure measurements by the station pull-through (SPT) technique are a little more difficult to determine. You will assess not only pressure but also the relaxation of the sphincter in response to a swallow. Before attempting a measurement, survey the completed SPT from the GBL pressure through the LES to esophageal pressure, noting relaxations, pressure variations, and the pressure inversion point (PIP) (Fig. 5.3). This will give you a general feel for the sphincter before doing the actual measurements. Complete relaxation with a swallow is demonstrated by a decrease to 0 mm Hg (GBL) with a duration of about 10 sec. Remember that a *normal* sphincter should always relax with a wet swallow (Fig. 5.4A). Stating that sphincter relaxation is abnormal based only on dry swallows is inaccurate.

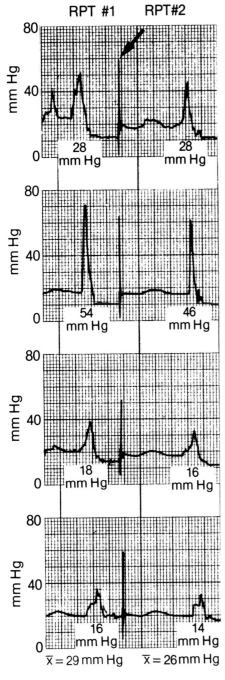

FIGURE 5.2 A series of two RPTs providing eight individual LES pressure measurements. Averaging the eight values represents the mean LES pressure. Arrow points to line resulting from pressure rise from reinsertion of catheter across the LES for second pull-through.

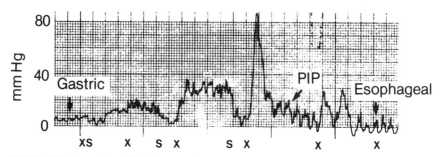

FIGURE 5.3 A completed SPT from the GBL, through the LES, to the body of the esophagus. Tube moved up at 0.5 cm intervals (x) and swallows (s) recorded at each interval.

Usually, however, even dry swallows will result in adequate sphincter relaxation. As with the RPT, four different measurements are made using the GBL as a 0-mm Hg reference point. The actual measurement is from the highest pressure zone or segment, but the reading will be taken *not* to the top of the tracing but to the *midpoint* of the respiratory variations. (Remember

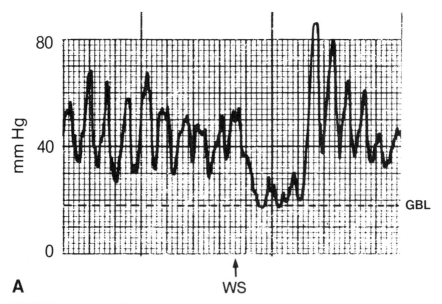

FIGURE 5.4A Normal LES relaxation to GBL after a wet swallow (ws).

that part of the variation in pressures seen in the SPT is due to respiration.) The highest midpoint is usually found immediately before the PIP. Measure from the midpoint of the respiratory variations to the GBL to find the LES pressure reading for that port (Fig. 5.4B). Make all four pressure determinations and average them for the LES pressure by the SPT technique. Do not base your measurements on a random, single, high peak, as this may be artifactual, but preferably from three to five stable respirations at a fixed station. The measurement should not be taken directly after a swallow-induced relaxation, since the resulting baseline pressure is often higher for a

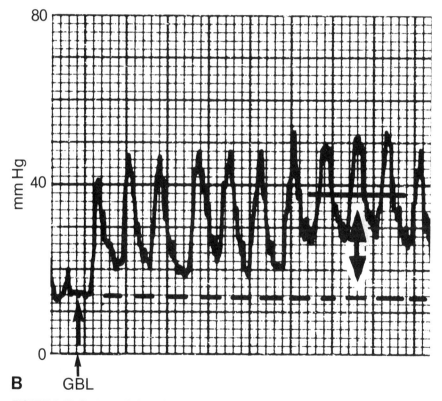

B   GBL

FIGURE 5.4B Station pull-through is measured from the highest midpoint of the respiratory variations to the GBL. At this point, SPT is 24 mm Hg. The numbers on the left refer to the range setting on the physiograph.

brief time (Fig. 5.5). This post-swallow high pressure becomes more pronounced as you enter the segment of the LES nearest the esophageal body. This is a result of the contraction in the body of the esophagus.

In the esophageal body, measurements of amplitude, duration, and velocity are made for peristaltic contractions following wet swallows. Special attention is directed to measurements made from the openings 3 and 8 cm above the LES, because esophageal motility disorders occur more frequently in the distal segment of the esophagus. Dry swallows or double swallows are not usually measured. Although nonperistaltic swallows are not measured, their presence is evaluated in determining the nature of the esophageal motility disorders. Do not select the "best" swallows. Try to assess ten contractions in sequence if possible.

Amplitude is a measurement of how tightly the muscles of the esophagus are squeezing during a contraction and is expressed in mm Hg. The baseline (0 mm Hg) is the pressure in the body of the esophagus between swallows. Contraction amplitude is measured from the baseline to the peak of the

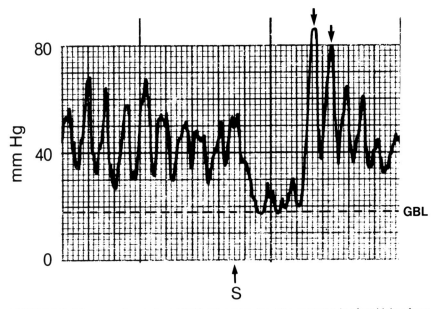

FIGURE 5.5 After a swallow-induced LES relaxation, baseline pressure is often higher for a brief time (arrows).

pressure wave (Fig. 5.6). After the amplitude of ten contractions in response to wet swallows has been measured, determine the mean value obtained from each orifice. Mean values from the 3- and 8-cm orifices can be averaged to obtain the *distal esophageal amplitude* (DEA).

   Duration is a measurement of how long, in seconds, the muscles of the esophagus are squeezing during a contraction. The measurement is made from the point where the upstroke of the contraction leaves the baseline to the point where the downstroke of the contraction comes back to the baseline (Fig. 5.7). The esophageal baseline sometimes rises before the actual contraction as a result of the ingested water bolus. In this situation, you may

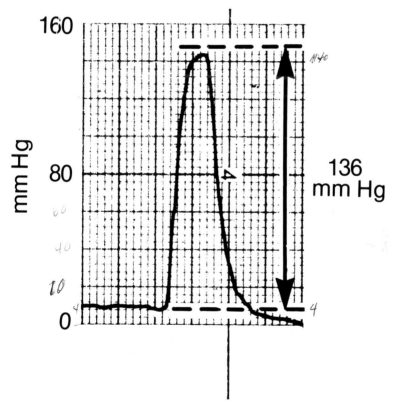

FIGURE 5.6 Contraction amplitude (mm Hg) is measured from the esophageal baseline to the peak of the pressure wave. The numbers on the left refer to the range setting on the physiograph.

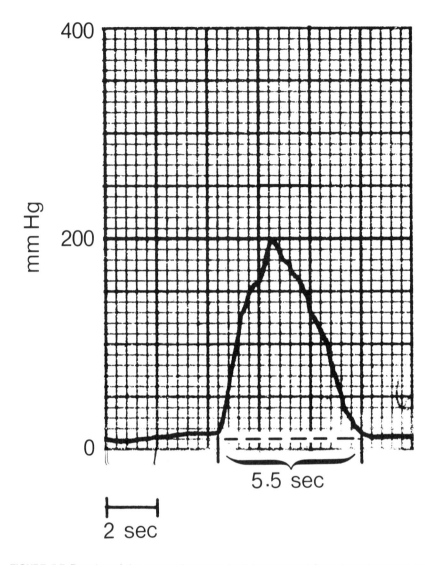

FIGURE 5.7 Duration of the contraction wave (sec) is measured from the point where the upstroke of the contraction leaves the baseline to the point where the downstroke comes back to the baseline. At a proper paper speed of 2.5 mm/sec, each large box represents 2 sec.

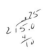

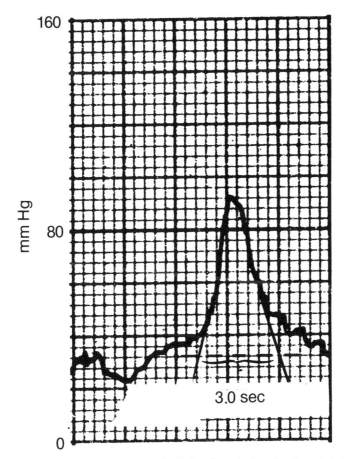

FIGURE 5.8 The esophageal baseline may rise before the actual contraction wave, as a result of the ingested water bolus. In this situation, you may need to extend the slope of the contraction wave to the baseline to better define the onset and termination of the contraction wave.

need to extend the slope of the contraction to the baseline and measure from that point (Fig. 5.8). Use a paper speed of 2.5 mm/sec during swallows.

Velocity may not be routinely determined, but it is important to know what it means and how to measure it. Velocity is a measurement of how fast the contraction wave moves down the esophagus. It is expressed in cm/sec. This measurement is made by determining the time between the beginning of the upstroke of the contractions at 13 and 3 cm above the LES. This time (in seconds) is then divided into 10, which is the number of centimeters between the ports at 13 and 3 cm (Fig. 5.9).

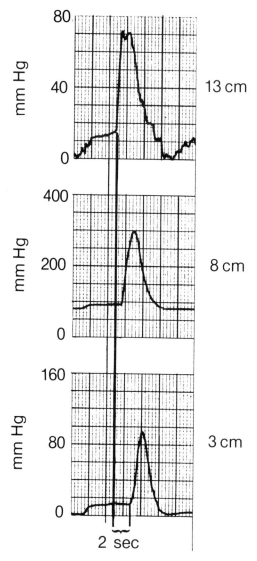

FIGURE 5.9 Velocity is measured by determining the time between the beginning of the upstroke of the contractions at 13 and 3 cm above the LES. In this example, the interval is 2 sec.

$$\text{Therefore, velocity} = \frac{10 \text{ cm}}{2 \text{ sec}} = 5 \text{ cm/sec.}$$

Paper speed is 2.5 mm/sec.

Double- and Triple-Peaked Contractions

Peristaltic contractions that have two pressure peaks are called double-peaked contractions and are considered a variant of normal contractions (Fig. 5.10). Contraction amplitude should be measured for the higher peak. Duration is measured from the upstroke of the first peak to the downstroke of the last.

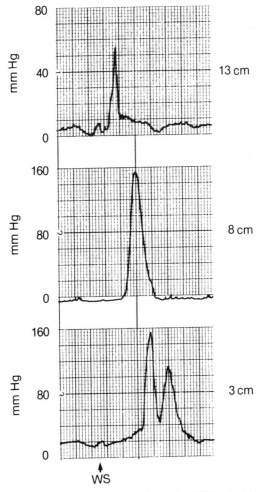

FIGURE 5.10 The contraction wave at 3 cm above the LES is double peaked. WS, wet swallow.

Triple-peaked peristaltic contractions are considered abnormal. Each peak should be at least 10% of the overall wave amplitude and 1 sec in duration (Fig. 5.11). Measure the amplitude and duration as for double-peaked waves.

Nonperistaltic Contractions

The occurrence of a nonperistaltic contraction following a wet swallow is usually abnormal. Simultaneous and retrograde contractions constitute nonperistaltic contractions. A simultaneous contraction indicates that large portions of the esophagus are contracting *at the same time*, instead of in the normal, peristaltic sequence. In some cases the entire esophagus contracts together while, in other cases, only the mid- or distal esophagus contracts

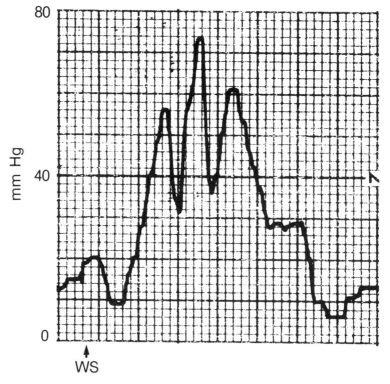

FIGURE 5.11 A triple-peaked contraction is considered abnormal. Each peak should be at least 10% of the overall wave amplitude and 1 sec in duration. WS, wet swallow.

simultaneously. Simultaneous contractions may be identical at adjacent sites (Fig. 5.12A) or may begin together and peak peristaltically (Fig. 5.12B). Retrograde contractions occur when the distal esophagus contracts *before* the proximal esophagus (Fig. 5.13).

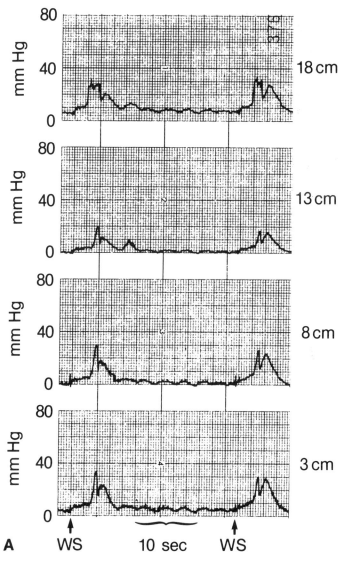

FIGURE 5.12A Two simultaneous contractions after wet swallows (WS). These contractions are identical in appearance at the three most distal recording ports (13, 8, and 3 cm).

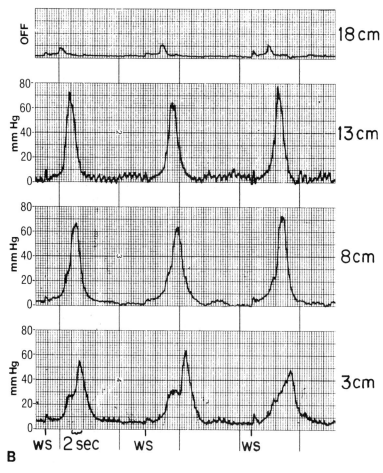

FIGURE 5.12B Series of three simultaneous contractions after wet swallows (WS). In the three most distal recording ports, the onset of the contractions are identical but peak peristaltically. Since the bolus is pushed along by the front of the contraction wave, the onset rather than peak of the contraction determines orderly peristaltic movement. Paper speed is 2.5 mm/sec.

Nontransmitted Contractions

Occasionally a wet swallow will be followed by *no* activity in the distal esophagus. This is known as a nontransmitted wave. A measurement of more than 20% nontransmitted waves after wet swallows is considered abnormal.

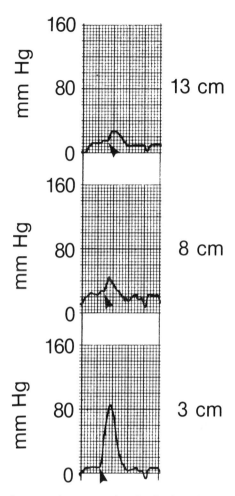

FIGURE 5.13 Retrograde contractions occur when the distal esophagus contracts before the proximal esophagus. In this example, the distal esophagus contracts 0.4 to 0.8 sec before the more proximal esophagus.

Spontaneous Contractions

A spontaneous contraction is a contraction of the body of the esophagus that is not initiated by a swallow. It may result from distention of the esophagus by material that was poorly cleared by a swallow or refluxed from the stomach. Spontaneous contractions may be recorded from one or multiple ports and be either peristaltic (secondary peristalsis) or simultaneous. These contractions are best seen during quiet periods with ad lib swallowing, because regular 30-sec swallow intervals interfere with the generation of spontaneous contractions.

Provocative Tests

Remember that the interpretation of the provocative tests is subjective and based on what the patients say they feel. No manometric measurements are made.

UPPER ESOPHAGEAL SPHINCTER

Upper esophageal sphincter measurements can be made from the esophageal baseline pressure to the pressure rise seen while the orifice is in the UES. Like the lower sphincter, the upper sphincter relaxes completely to baseline pressure with a swallow. After the UES relaxation, the muscles briefly contract more tightly than before, causing a rise in pressure on the tracing. This is known as the post-relaxation augmentation (Fig. 5.14). To assess the coordi-

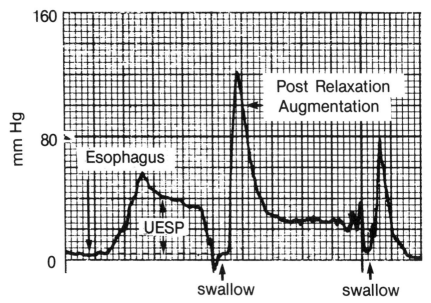

FIGURE 5.14 Upper esophageal sphincter pressure (UESP) is measured from baseline esophageal pressure to steady-state pressure obtained while the orifice is in the UES. After UES relaxation, the muscles briefly contract more tightly than before causing a rise in pressure — the post-relaxation augmentation.

nation of the pharyngeal contraction with the relaxation of the UES, the first port (most proximal) on the catheter must clear the UES and be in the pharynx while the second port is in the UES. The patient is asked to swallow, and coordination is assessed by comparing the timing sequence between the spike of the pharyngeal contraction and the UES relaxation. Peak pharyngeal pressures normally occur during the trough of UES relaxation (Fig. 5.15). This assessment is subsequently repeated, as the last two ports are positioned in the UES. If a motility disorder of the UES is suspected, several wet and dry swallows should be obtained as the three more distal ports pass through the UES.

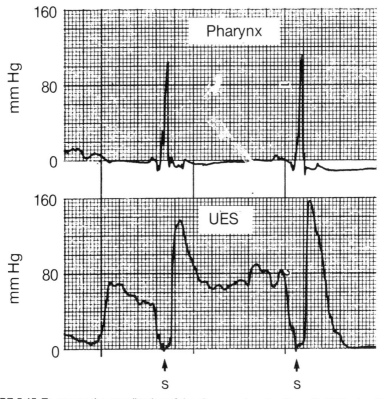

FIGURE 5.15 To assess the coordination of the pharyngeal contraction with UES relaxation, the proximal port must be in the pharynx while the second port is in the UES. Normally, in response to a swallow(s), peak pharyngeal pressures occur during the trough of UES relaxation.

Patient:_____ Date:_____

Age:_____ Service:_____

Unit #:_____ Prior UGI surgery:_____

Tracing #:_____ Phone number:_____

Address:_____

HISTORY:

Heartburn_____ Dysphagia_____ Odynophagia_____

Chest pain_____ Nausea_____ Vomiting_____

Regurgitation_____ Night cough_____ Asthma_____

OTHERS:

Cardiac cath./work-up

Radiology:

Endoscopy:

MANOMETRY REPORT:

Upper esophageal sphincter (UES):

Esophageal body:

Lower esophageal sphincter (LES):

Bernstein's test

Edrophonium test (mg)

IMPRESSIONS:

FIGURE 5.16 Esophageal manometry report.

FINAL REPORT

The final report form (Fig. 5.16) should include all measurements and values derived from the esophageal manometry study. It should also indicate the results of any provocative testing. A diagnosis and possible treatment should be included under the impressions section.

CHAPTER 6

Normal Values
for Esophageal Manometry

Joel E. Richter, MD, FACP

As the field of esophageal motility has moved from an art to a scientifically based area of investigation, it has become increasingly important to define the range of normal values for esophageal pressures. Recent technical advancements, particularly the use of low-compliance pneumohydraulic infusion pumps and miniature intraesophageal pressure transducers now allow accurate pressure measurements from the esophageal body as well as from the lower esophageal sphincter (LES).[1] Increasing clinical and investigative use of esophageal manometry has also improved our recognition of esophageal motility abnormalities. Fifteen years ago, achalasia and diffuse esophageal spasm were the only commonly recognized motility disorders. Today, the gastroenterologist must also be able to identify the nutcracker esophagus (high-amplitude peristaltic contractions in the distal esophagus), hypertensive LES, motility abnormalities associated with collagen vascular diseases, and a number of miscellaneous abnormalities grouped under the broad term *nonspecific esophageal motility disorders*. To better appreciate these newer, more subtle esophageal motility abnormalities, we must have a strong database to define our normal esophageal pressure values.

PRIOR STUDIES

The LES was first identified manometrically by Fyke and associates in 1956.[2] For the next fifteen years, investigative interests focused on this sphincter and its difference in healthy subjects and patients with gastro-esophageal reflux. Critical interest in pressures along the esophageal body only began in the mid-1970s with the introduction of low-compliance infusion pumps. Before the newer technology, a contraction pressure of more than 40 to 50 mm Hg was considered to be of abnormally high amplitude.[3] Initial studies primarily focused attention on younger subjects, with mean ages in the twenties,[4,5] or the very elderly.[6] Small study populations (usually less than 25 subjects) also limited these earlier observations. Studies by Dodds et al[4] and Hollis and Castell[5] were instrumental in defining the differences in pressures and peristaltic activity induced by dry versus wet swallows. The latter investigators were also the first to suggest that age may alter esophageal contraction pressures.[6] They observed a marked decline in the amplitude of contraction waves for subjects older than 80 years, possibly the result of age-related weakening in esophageal smooth muscle. More recently, Clouse and Staiano have reported manometric data from 40 healthy volunteers with a mean age of 40 ± 2.8 ($\pm$ SE) years.[7] Although they investigated a larger group of subjects, their data analysis did not permit separation of the effects of age on contraction parameters. In our laboratory, we have recently completed a large study of 95 healthy subjects, using the best available manometric techniques to better define the normal range of esophageal pressures and activity.[8] Particular attention was given to adult volunteers between 40 and 70 years old, because these are the ages when patients present with unexplained noncardiac chest pain, which is possibly related to esophageal dysfunction.

NORMAL VALUES BASED ON OUR EXPERIENCE IN 95 HEALTHY VOLUNTEERS

Study Population and Manometry Methods

This study included 95 volunteers with a mean age of 43 ± 2.5 ($\pm$ SE) years and an age range of 22 to 79 years. There were 38 men and 59 women. Their age distribution, according to decades, was as follows: twenties, 22 subjects; thirties, 20 subjects; forties, 20 subjects; fifties, 20 subjects; and sixties or older, 13 subjects. The sex distribution in all decades was similar to the overall group. Volunteers were excluded if there was a history of frequent heartburn (more than once a month), dysphagia for either solids or liquids, regurgitation, chest pain, or antacid use. Additionally, no volunteer had a history of esophageal surgery, diabetes mellitus, collagen vascular disease, or neurologic disorder. Medication histories were closely reviewed and no volunteer was taking any drugs known to alter esophageal function at the time of the study.

Esophageal manometry was performed by the techniques described in Chapter 4. All studies were done with a round 8-lumen polyvinyl catheter (diameter 4.5 mm; Arndorfer Specialties, Inc., Greendale, WI) and low-compliance pneumohydraulic capillary-infusion system (Arndorfer Specialties, Inc.). LES pressures were measured by both the rapid (RPT) and station (SPT) pull-through techniques. Contractions in the esophageal body were measured with the four proximal openings positioned 3, 8, 13, and 18 cm above the LES. Fifteen wet swallows (5 cc of water) were given, separated by 30-sec intervals. The first five swallows were used as a training period to adapt the subjects to the technique and therefore only the last ten swallows were analyzed. The wet swallows were then followed by ten dry swallows, separated by 30-sec intervals, and a 5-min quiet period, used to evaluate spontaneous esophageal activity. During the quiet period, the subjects were instructed to relax, not talk, and dry swallow only as necessary.

The parameters of the pressure wave (amplitude, duration, velocity) as well as the percentage of "abnormal" contractions (nonperistaltic contractions including simultaneous and nontransmitted swallows, double- and triple-peaked waves, retrograde contraction sequences, and spontaneous contractions) were defined and measured as described in Chapter 5. Individual values for the recording sites at 3 and 8 cm above the LES were also combined and designated as distal esophageal contraction pressures, since recent evidence suggests that most esophageal motility abnormalities are confined to this region of the esophagus.[7]

Parameters of the Pressure Wave

Amplitude

The mean amplitude of the contraction waves recorded from the four esophageal sites in our 95 volunteers is shown in Table 6.1. Amplitude increases distally along the esophagus. Mean distal esophageal amplitude (DEA) for contractions after wet swallows 99 ± 40 mm Hg (± 1 SD). As has been previously reported,[4,5,9] mean contraction amplitude is significantly greater ($P < 0.001$) for wet swallows than for dry swallows at all recording sites.

Contraction amplitude is found to vary with age after wet swallows but not dry swallows. Mean DEA (Fig. 6.1), as well as mean amplitude at 3 and 8 cm above the LES, increases with each decade to a peak in the fifties. The data indicate that the mean DEA for the subjects in their fifties and forties is significantly greater ($P < 0.05$) than the mean DEA for subjects in their twenties. Proximal contraction amplitudes do not vary with age and mean contraction amplitudes are similar for men and women of the same age.

TABLE 6.1 Esophageal Pressure Data for Normal Subjects

Recording Site (cm above LES)	Wet Swallows	Dry Swallows	P Value[a]
Amplitude (mm Hg; $\bar{x} \pm 1$ SD)			
18	62 ± 29	44 ± 25	<0.001
13	70 ± 32	48 ± 27	<0.001
8	90 ± 41	63 ± 32	<0.001
3	109 ± 45	79 ± 33	<0.001
3/8 (DEA)	99 ± 40	71 ± 28	<0.001
Duration (sec; $\bar{x} \pm 1$ SD)			
18	2.8 ± 0.8	2.6 ± 0.7	NS[b]
13	3.5 ± 0.7	3.4 ± 0.6	NS
8	3.9 ± 0.9	3.8 ± 0.8	NS
3	4.0 ± 1.1	4.2 ± 0.8	NS
3/8 (DED)	3.9 ± 0.9	4.1 ± 0.8	NS
Velocity (cm/sec; $\bar{x} \pm 1$ SD)			
Proximal	3.0 ± 0.6	4.0 ± 0.4	<0.001
Distal	3.5 ± 0.9	4.0 ± 0.3	<0.001
Lower Esophageal Sphincter Pressure ($\bar{x} \pm 1$ SD)			
RPT	29.0 ± 12.1		
SPT	24.4 ± 10.1		

[a]P value for peristaltic parameters obtained with wet versus dry swallows.
[b]NS, not significant.

These values for normal peristaltic contraction amplitude ($\bar{x} \pm 2$ SD) are considerably greater than previously reported. Two important factors may contribute to these differences. We used a larger, commercially available manometry catheter (4.5-mm diameter), as opposed to the catheter employed in prior studies (usually $\leq$ 3.3-mm diameter). Increases in catheter diameter cause significant increases in contraction amplitude as well as LES pressures.[10,11] This phenomenon is the result of the length–tension characteristics of esophageal smooth muscle, whereby increased stretch causes greater contractile forces. We have also studied a group of subjects older than those previously studied. The twenty-year-old volunteers studied in our laboratory have mean contraction amplitudes similar to earlier studies.[4,5] The significantly greater amplitudes in the older volunteers, however, accounted for the group's overall higher mean-contraction amplitude. This effect of age on the contraction amplitude is important to recognize and

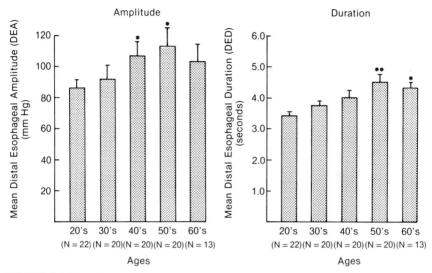

FIGURE 6.1 The effects of age on distal esophageal contraction pressures in 95 healthy volunteers. Mean DEA and DED of contractions after wet swallows increases with age and peaks in the fifties. Vertical lines indicate ± 1 SE. N, number of subjects in each group; *, $P<0.05$ compared to twenties; **, $P<0.05$ compared to twenties and thirties.

requires that higher upper limits be set in order to encompass the older patients frequently referred to the manometry laboratory. A more appropriate cutoff for the upper limit of normal should therefore be at least in excess of 180 mm Hg (Fig. 6.2).

Duration

The mean duration of the contraction waves recorded from the four esophageal sites in our 95 volunteers are shown in Table 6.1. Mean duration parallels amplitude by increasing distally along the esophagus. Despite this similar trend, poor correlation between individual amplitudes and durations is found for both wet ($r = 0.53$) and dry ($r = 0.55$) swallows. There is also no significant difference between mean contraction duration after wet or dry swallows at any recording site. Earlier studies[4,5] had suggested that the duration of the peristaltic pressure complex after wet swallows was greater than after dry swallows, but our findings and those of a more recent study[9] do not agree with this observation.

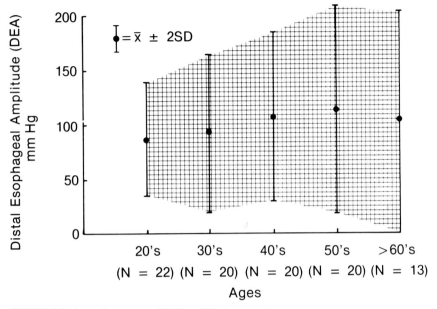

FIGURE 6.2 Values for mean ± 2 SD for DEA of contractions after wet swallows by decade in 95 healthy volunteers. The upper limits of the normal range increases linearly with age and peaks in the fifties. N, number of subjects in each decade.

As with amplitude, age has an important effect on duration after wet but not dry swallows. Mean distal esophageal duration (DED) for contractions, as well as mean duration at 3 and 8 cm above the LES, increases with each decade and peaks in the fifties (Fig. 6.1). The mean DED for the subjects in their fifties is significantly greater ($P < 0.05$) than the mean DED for subjects in their twenties and thirties. Mean DED for subjects in their sixties or older is also significantly greater ($P < 0.05$) than that found in the 20-year-old volunteers. Mean contraction duration is similar in men and women of the same age.

Velocity

In agreement with prior studies[4,5] both proximal and distal esophageal velocity were found to be significantly faster ($P < 0.001$) after dry compared to wet swallows (Table 6.1). Distal esophageal velocity is also significantly faster ($P < 0.01$) than proximal esophageal velocity after both types of swallow stimulus. Age and sex has no effect on esophageal velocity.

Lower Esophageal Sphincter Pressure

Mean LES pressure measured by RPT for the 95 volunteers in our laboratory is 29.0 ± 12.1 mm Hg (± 1 SD). Mean LES pressure measured by SPT in these same subjects is 24.4 ± 10.1 mm Hg at midrespiration (Table 6.1). As has been previously documented,[12,13] LES pressures are greater on the average when measured with the RPT as compared to the SPT technique. The correlation between the two methods, however, is not very strong ($r = 0.70$) and is indicative of the well-known minute-to-minute variability of measured pressures in the LES.[14] Age and sex had no effect on LES pressures measured by either technique.

"Abnormal" Motor Responses
Double- and Triple-Peaked Waves

Double-peaked waves are relatively common in normal subjects, occurring after 11% to 18% of swallows (Table 6.2). In individual subjects, the frequency of double-peaked waves ranges from 0%–90%. Double-peaked waves are characterized by prolonged duration [7.2 ± 1.0 sec (± SE)] and were confined to the two most distal recording sites. Neither age nor the type of swallow stimulus has any effect on the prevalence of double-peaked waves. Thus, double-peaked waves are a variant of normal waves and not absolutely diagnostic of diabetes with neuropathy, as recently reported by Loo et al.[15]

Triple-peaked waves, however, are rare. They occur after 0.1% of wet swallows and 0.3% of dry swallows, ie, one different person in each group was observed to have a single triple-peaked wave. This observation provides considerable support for the conclusion that triple-peaked contraction waves are an indication of an esophageal motility disorder.[7]

Nonperistaltic Contractions

As shown in Table 6.2, the prevalence of nonperistaltic contractions after dry swallows (18%) is significantly greater ($P < 0.001$) than after wet swallows (4%). This is not a new observation, as older studies have reported nonperistaltic contractions after 15%–29% of dry swallows and 3%–4% of wet swallows.[4,5] The difference in response to the two types of swallow stimulus is composed primarily of the significantly greater ($P < 0.001$) percentage of simultaneous contractions obtained after dry swallows (12%) compared to wet swallows (<1%) (Table 6.2). Thirty-seven percent of normal subjects in

TABLE 6.2 "Abnormal" Motor Responses for Normal Subjects[a]

	Double-Peaked Waves	Non-Peristaltic Contractions	Simultaneous Contractions	Non-transmitted Contractions	Retrograde Contractions
Wet swallows	11.3 ± 18.7 NS[b]	4.1 ± 8.3 $P < 0.001$	0.4 ± 2.0 $P < 0.001$	3.7 ± 8.0 NS	0 NS
Dry swallows	18.1 ± 19.4	18.1 ± 25.7	12.6 ± 23.5	5.5 ± 12.7	0

[a] Percentage of swallows ($\bar{x}$ ± 1 SD).
[b] NS, not significant.

our laboratory have at least one simultaneous contraction during a series of ten dry swallows, but only 4% have simultaneous contractions with wet swallows. The latter group represents four subjects, who each had one simultaneous contraction during a series of ten wet swallows. Two normal subjects were observed to have 80% and 100% of their dry swallows followed by simultaneous contractions, while all wet swallows were followed by peristaltic contractions (Fig. 6.3). This message carries considerable clinical importance, since abnormal motility, particularly diffuse esophageal spasm, may be overdiagnosed if dry rather than wet swallows are used to assess peristalsis. These results also support recent studies that redefine diffuse esophageal spasm based on the presence of greater than 10% simultaneous contractions after wet swallows in association with intermittent normal peristalsis (see Chapter 9).

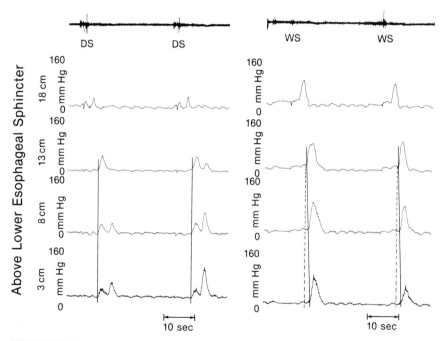

FIGURE 6.3 Manometry tracing showing a comparison of esophageal contractions after dry and wet swallows in the same healthy volunteer. As shown on the left, all dry swallows (DS) are followed by nonperistaltic simultaneous distal contractions. In contraction, as shown on the right, all wet swallows (WS) are followed by orderly peristaltic contractions. Also note that overall contractile amplitude at each recording site is greater for wet compared to dry swallows and that there are frequent double-peaked waves after dry swallows.

Spontaneous Contractions

During the 5-min quiet period, 19 out of 38 (50%) normal subjects were observed to have spontaneous activity not associated with dry swallows. These contractions are usually of low amplitude (30 to 60 mm Hg) and often simultaneous. The frequency of spontaneous contractions ranges from one per 5-min period to many simultaneous, repetitive contractions resembling diffuse esophageal spasm (Fig. 6.4). This observation suggests that frequent spontaneous activity may be a variation of normal contractions and must be interpreted cautiously in the diagnosis of diffuse esophageal spasm.[16]

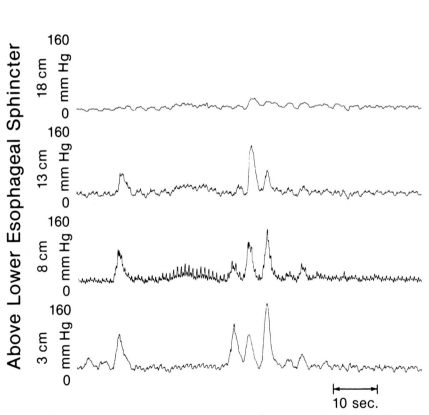

FIGURE 6.4 In healthy volunteers, spontaneous contractions are usually of low amplitude and often simultaneous. Occasionally, as shown here, these spontaneous contractions can be very frequent and resemble diffuse esophageal spasm.

CONCLUSION

We recommended that our normal esophageal motility database can be used in laboratories employing similar equipment, techniques, and analysis methods. We believe that our method of performing esophageal manometry has broad application to both the busy clinical practice and the research laboratory. The infusion pumps, transducers, and catheters used in our studies are all standardized and commercially available. Our station method, used for mapping the esophageal body, is more easily performed than the centimeter-by-centimeter pull-through method and requires less than 10 minutes. Data analysis is also faster for ten swallows than the 30 or more swallows recommended for the pull-through method.[7] Regardless of method, the state of the art now suggests that esophageal pressures and peristalsis need to be evaluated by wet swallows. Dry swallows have no place in the modern day diagnosis of esophageal motility disorders.

REFERENCES

1. Dodds WJ: Instrumentation and methods for intraluminal esophageal manometry. *Arch Intern Med* 1976;136:515–523.
2. Fyke FE, Code CF, Schlegal JF: The gastroesophageal sphincter in healthy humans. *Gastroenterologia* 1956;86:135–150.
3. Nagler R, Spiro HM: Serial esophageal motility studies in asymptomatic young subjects. *Gastroenterology* 1961;41:371–379.
4. Dodds WJ, Hogan WJ, Reid DP, et al: A comparison between primary esophageal peristalsis following wet and dry swallows. *J Appl Physiol* 1973;35:851–857.
5. Hollis JB, Castell DO: Effect of dry swallows and wet swallows of different volumes of esophageal peristalsis. *J Appl Physiol* 1975;38:1161–1164.
6. Hollis JB, Castell DO: Esophageal function in elderly men. A new look at "presby-esophagus." *Ann Intern Med* 1974;80:371–374.
7. Clouse RE, Staiano A: Contraction abnormalities of the esophageal body in patients referred for manometry: a new approach to manometric classification. *Dig Dis Sci* 1983; 28:784–791.
8. Richter JE, Wu WC, Johns DN, et al: Esophageal manometry in 95 healthy adult volunteers: variability of pressure with age and frequency of "abnormal" contractions. *Dig Dis Sci* (in press).
9. Kaye MD, Wexler RM: Alteration of esophageal peristalsis by body position. *Dig Dis Sci* 1981;26:897–901.
10. Kaye MD, Showalter JP: Measurement of pressure in the lower esophageal sphincter. The influence of catheter diameter. *Dig Dis Sci* 1974;19:860–863.
11. Lydon SB, Dodds WJ, Hogan WJ, et al: The effect of manometric assembly diameter on intraluminal esophageal pressure recording. *Dig Dis Sci* 1975;20:968–970.
12. Dodds WJ, Hogan WJ, Stef JJ, et al: A rapid pull-through technique for measuring lower esophageal sphincter pressure. *Gastroenterology* 1975;68:437–442.

13. Welch RW, Drake ST: Normal lower esophageal sphincter: a comparison of rapid vs. slow pull-through techniques. *Gastroenterology* 1980;78:1446–1451.
14. Dent J, Dodds WJ, Friedman RH, et al: Mechanism of gastroesophageal reflux in recumbent asymptomatic healthy subjects. *J Clin Invest* 1980;65:256–267.
15. Loo FD, Dodds WJ, Soergel KH, et al: Multipeaked esophageal peristaltic pressure waves in patients with diabetic neuropathy. *Gastroenterology* 1985;88:485–491.
16. Gilles M, Nick R, Skyring A: Clinical, manometrics and pathological studies in diffuse esophageal spasm. *Br Med J* 1967;2:527–530.

CHAPTER 7

The Computer
in the Motility Laboratory

June A. Castell, MS

INTRODUCTION

Recent advances in computer technology, particularly the reduction in both the size of the equipment and its cost, along with an increase in capability, have made the use of the computer in the motility laboratory an attractive prospect. There are several valid reasons for developing a computer capability. First is the attendant increase in accuracy; voltages are read directly. This means that one does not have to allow for variation in either line width or zero settings. Baseline irregularities can be compensated for with smoothing techniques. Second, computer analysis not only increases accuracy, it decreases variability. Parameters are read using the same algorithm each time. Variations and approximations used in the manual extrapolation of endpoints are eliminated. Since motility studies are generally concerned with changes in parameters, consistency is particularly important. Third, computers are capable of saving time in the motility laboratory. About 1 hour is required to read and obtain mean values of a normal tracing of ten wet swallows. The computer analysis of this same tracing takes about 10 minutes and is completed by the time the technician has the patient off the table. No additional technician or physician time is required to analyze the tracing. This becomes increasingly significant as the number of studies done increases. The reduction in physician or technician time also represents a saving of money. Again, this is significant only if a large number of studies is done. In fact, time and money savings are really secondary to the advantages gained in accuracy and decreased variability. Lastly, computer analysis of motility studies also provides the capability to analyze parameters that are difficult or impossible to determine manually.

Criteria for a Successful Motility Laboratory Computer

The term "computer" without modifiers encompasses such a large family of equipment that it is almost meaningless. At this time our motility laboratory has successfully been computerized using a standard microcomputer or "personal computer." It is small and will easily and unobstrusively fit into the normal laboratory environment. Personal computers are readily available and relatively inexpensive. Parts are also readily available and it is usually easy to find competent and prompt service organizations. They are easy for the lay person to learn to operate and are relatively easy to program. However, the successful motility laboratory computer must be capable of direct online analysis. This means that a standard microcomputer must be augmented with an analog to digital (A/D) capability and it must have sufficient internal memory and data storage to accommodate a normal motility study. In addition, it must not require specialized technical skills to operate, as it most certainly will be operated by the technician or physician doing the study. It must also be unobstrusive and not delay or otherwise impact the study. It must allow for interactions between the computer and the investigator to allow for manual control of the direction of the study and, of course, the successful motility laboratory computer must analyze motility tracings at least as well as a human, and it must do so in a timely and cost-effective way.

In the gastrointestinal (GI) section at the Bowman Gray School of Medicine, we have been experimenting with the computerization of our motility laboratory for about two years. The equipment that we have been using is shown in Figure 7.1. It includes an Apple IIE microcomputer with 64K internal memory and two external floppy disk drives. This basic configuration is augmented with an ADALAB (Interactive Microwave, Inc.) A/D converter and a fast A/D multiplexer. We also use a standard Epson printer with graphics capability. One of the primary reasons for the selection of this particular configuration was the commercial availability of an ASSEMBLY language program for A/D sampling. This program is addressable through higher-level languages and has simple commands for software selection of channel, rate of collection, length of collection, and voltage-gain settings. A total system was developed by incorporating this ASSEMBLY language program into a main program written in BASIC. The BASIC program allows interaction between the computer and the investigator, so that criteria for

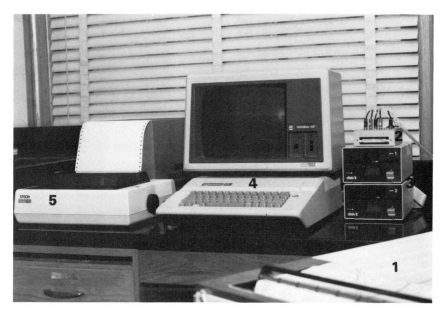

FIGURE 7.1 Equipment used for computer interface of online esophageal motility analysis. (1) Chart recorder; (2) connector box transmitting output from the recorder to the A/D board in the computer; (3) dual floppy-disk drives; (4) Apple IIE computer; (5) Epson printer.

individual experiments can be established. Upon a signal from the investigator, control is automatically passed to the ASSEMBLY language program for sampling the data channels. The computer collects from these channels a discrete numeric equivalent of a continuous voltage at a predetermined sampling rate. Once these voltages have been collected they are converted to mm Hg via an algorithm which was derived from an independent calibration of the A/D board with a mercury manometer applied to the external transducers. Since the data points are collected at a predetermined and constant rate, each data point represents not only a specific pressure but also a specific time. Once these data points are collected and converted to mm Hg, the data can be analyzed for all pertinent parameters. Independent parameter values and mean values are then reported.

In order to verify that the computer has met the criterion that it can analyze motility tracings at least as well as a human, two separate experiments were conducted. In the first, ten wet swallows and lower esophageal sphincter (LES) pressure [rapid pull-through (RPT) technique] were ana-

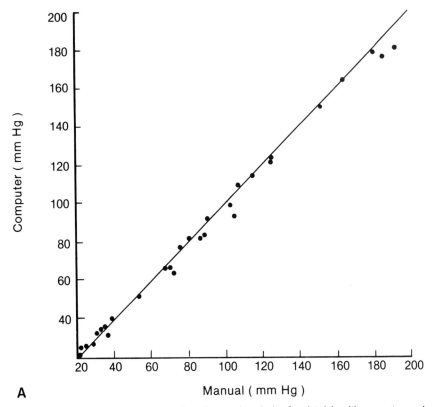

A

FIGURE 7.2 Graphs showing correlation of manual analysis of peristalsis with computer analysis for **(A)** amplitude ($r = 0.99$), **(B)** duration ($r = 0.83$), and **(C)** velocity ($r = 0.89$). Solid line represents line of identity and broken line represents calculated regression line.

lyzed by computer. The tracings were then read by five different individuals, each experienced in the interpretation of manometric tracings. The means of the five sets of manually determined values for all peristalsis parameters were compared to the computer-derived values, using standard correlation and regression analysis techniques. The results are shown in Figure 7.2. The second experiment was similar, except that the LES pressure was found by the station pull-through (SPT) technique and sphincter relaxation parameters were measured during wet and dry swallows. These results are shown in Figure 7.3.

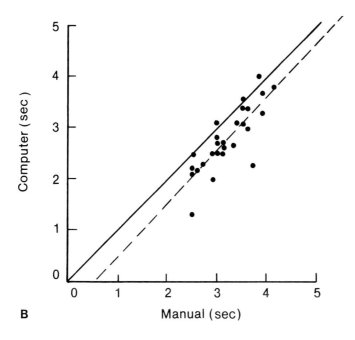

B

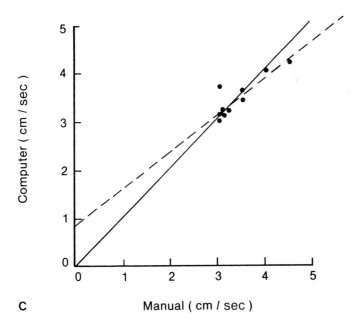

C

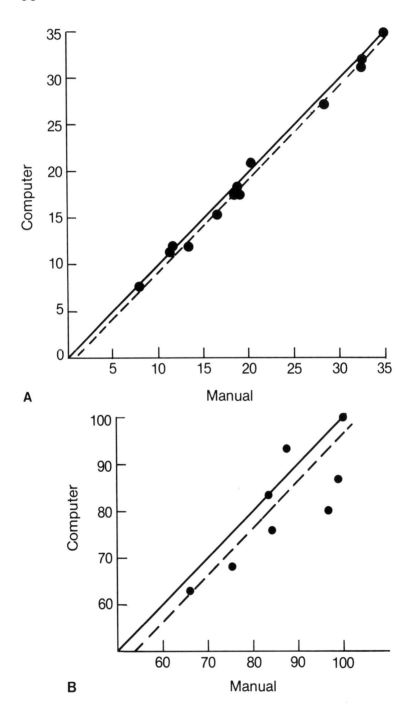

A

B

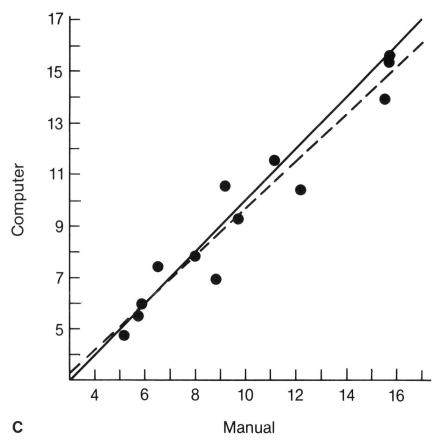

FIGURE 7.3 Graphs illustrating correlation between manual and computer interpretation of LES relaxation. The parameters measured include **(A)** resting LES pressure (mm Hg; $y = -0.82 + x$; $r = 0.99$), **(B)** percent LES relaxation ($y = -4.7 + 1.01x$; $r = 0.87$), and **(C)** duration of LES relaxation (sec; $y = 0.43 + 0.9x$; $r = 0.96$). Solid line represents line of identity and broken line represents calculated regression line.

Analysis of Wave Parameters during Peristalsis

Peristalsis is usually analyzed by sampling pressures at three locations within the body of the esophagus during a swallow. Commonly, the most distal of these measurements is made at 3–5 cm above the lower esophageal sphincter with the mid- and proximal measurements made at 5-cm intervals. Figure 7.4 is a diagram of the kind of pressure profile one normally sees, and

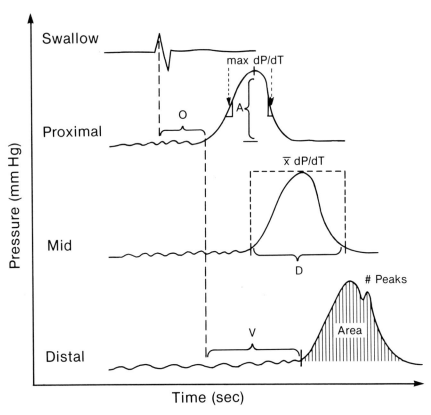

FIGURE 7.4 Schematic representation of parameters of the peristaltic wave measured by the computer. O, time between onset of swallow and beginning of peristaltic wave at each recording site; A, amplitude of peristaltic wave; D, duration of peristaltic wave; V, velocity of peristaltic wave measured from the onset of the proximal to the onset of the distal wave.

we will use it to define the parameters that we are interested in analyzing. The amplitude, duration, mean and maximum slopes *(dP/dT)*, both up and down, the area under the wave, and the number of peaks are determined for each location. The velocity of the wave as it moves down the esophagus is also calculated. The onset of a swallow is indicated by changing the signal on a constantly monitored channel from low to high. This can be done either manually or by a change in pressure, as recorded by a pneumograph attached around the pharynx. Once the swallow is begun, data is collected on three channels for 15 sec. A baseline pressure is calculated for each channel by averaging the data points collected during the first 2 sec. Averaging is done in order to smooth out respiratory variations. The amplitudes are determined by finding the highest pressure during the collection period and subtracting the baseline pressure. The duration is determined by locating the beginning and the end of the wave. This is done by working from the peak outward in both directions to the first value less than the baseline plus 10 mm Hg. Waves of less than 10 mm Hg above the baseline are considered to be nontransmitted and are reported as such. Since the position in the data collection array of the identified pressures defines the time that that data point was collected, the duration can be defined as the difference in collection times between the last point and the first point identified, as described above. Wave durations significantly shorter (ie, less than 2 sec) than normally expected are annotated in the report and the investigator is advised to check the tracing for possible artifacts (cough, sneeze, etc). This algorithm for computing wave duration, that is, locating the beginning and the end of the wave at 10 mm Hg above the baseline, results in a slightly shorter duration than that which is normally measured manually. However, this algorithm was chosen to avoid baseline artifacts, such as a low-level pressure plateau preceding the wave itself. Since manometric studies are primarily interested in changes in duration, consistency in measurement is more important than the actual method. Mean slope is calculated as the change in pressure (ie, the peak amplitude minus the baseline) divided by the time from the beginning of the wave to the time of the wave peak *(dP/dT* up) or by the time from the peak to the end of the wave *(dP/dT* down). Maximum slope is determined by calculating the change in pressure over time in overlapping ⅓-sec segments from the beginning to the peak and from the peak to the end of the wave. Sign differences differentiate *dP/dT* up from *dP/dT* down. The area under the wave is calculated as the integral of the pressure values from the beginning to the end of the wave. The wave velocity is defined as the distance between the proximal and distal recording sites (10 cm) divided by elapsed time from the beginning of the proximal wave to the beginning of the distal wave. Wave velocity is also calculated as the distance between the proximal and distal recording sites divided by the elapsed time from the peak of the proximal wave to the peak of the distal wave. Wave velocities of greater than 10 cm/sec are considered simultaneous and are reported as such. The number of peaks is found by moving down the wave from the main peak (ie, highest recorded pressure), in both directions in overlapping ⅓-sec segments, looking for inflection points or places where the slope changes sign. In order to avoid calling artifacts "peaks," two additional criteria are applied: (1) a secondary peak must have an amplitude of at least 10% that of the primary peak and (2) it must endure for at least 1 sec.

At the conclusion of the analysis, a report showing the computer-determined values in all parameters for each of three waves for all swallows is printed. An example of this report is shown in Figure 7.5. A second report, giving mean values for all parameters for each wave, may also be generated.

```
This is swallow 9

This is the Distal Wave
The Total Number of Peaks is              1
The Peak Amplitude is                     181 mm Hg
The Wave Duration is                      3.4 sec
The Beginning of the Wave is              5.67 sec
The Average Upstroke, dP/dT, is           150.9 mm Hg/sec
The (dP/dT)/P Ratio is                    .96
The Maximum Upstroke, dP/dT, is           174 mm Hg/sec
The Average Downstroke, dP/dT, is         82.2 mm Hg/sec
The Maximum Downstroke, dP/dT, is         141 mm Hg/sec
The Wave Area is                          4247

The Wave Velocity is                      3.57 cm/sec
The Peak to Peak Velocity is              4.05
```

FIGURE 7.5 Example of computer printout of parameters analyzed for a single wave during a single swallow.

The system itself makes no clinical judgements based on the analysis of the peristaltic wave. It does, however, provide the investigator with some options and messages by highlighting possible abnormal situations. The investigator may exclude from the analysis any swallow that is considered unsatisfactory. A wave duration of less than 2 sec is quite unusual and may, in fact, represent an artifact. Therefore, durations of less than 2 sec are flagged with a warning message and the investigator is advised to refer to the tracing for verification. If the wave velocity exceeds 10 mm/sec, the wave is considered simultaneous and is so noted on the report. Simultaneous waves are not averaged into the mean velocities for a series of swallows. This, too, is noted on the report. Low-amplitude waves may include artifacts as multiple peaks. Waves with three or more peaks are annotated with a warning message that more than two peaks is considered abnormal. Waves of less than 10 mm of Hg are considered nontransmitted, are not averaged into the mean amplitudes for a series of swallows, and are so annotated on the report.

Analysis of Lower Esophageal Sphincter Pressures and Relaxation

Lower esophagus sphincter pressures are analyzed by two quite different techniques. In the RPT technique, four orifices at the same level, oriented 90° radially, are pulled rapidly from the stomach, through the sphincter, and into the esophagus. This passage through the sphincter is recorded on each of four channels as a separate pressure peak. Pull-through is normally done twice and the LES pressure is calculated as the mean of eight such pressure peaks. Computer analysis includes measuring a gastric baseline pressure on each of four channels for 1 sec and finding the mean. Data points are then collected on the four channels for 10 sec and the highest pressures are located. Sphincter pressures represent the high pressures minus the baseline pressures. The system allows the investigator to do up to four rapid pull-throughs and to select those two considered best.

The second technique for measuring LES pressures is the station pull-through (SPT). In this technique, an orifice is positioned in the stomach and pulled slowly into the sphincter measuring pressures at ½-cm intervals. Once the high-pressure zone is located, the orifice is left there and sphincter function during swallowing can be analyzed. Again, the computer system that analyzes lower esophageal sphincter (LES) function is set up as a dialog between the computer and the investigator so that the investigator can select such experimental parameters as number of swallows and gain settings. With the orifice in the stomach, gastric pressure is measured for 10 sec and then averaged to smooth out respiratory variations. Lower esophageal sphincter baseline pressure is measured for 15 sec and averaged to smooth out respiratory variations. The longer sampling period is due to greater respiratory variations within the sphincter. The LES pressure is then reported as the baseline pressure minus the gastric pressure. The sphincter relaxation phase is measured for 20 sec after the initiation of the swallow. The parameters of interest are shown in Figure 7.6. The relaxation is considered to have begun once the pressure drops below the *lowest* point obtained during the baseline

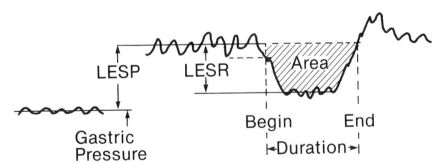

FIGURE 7.6 Schematic representation of parameters measured during computer analysis of lower esophageal sphincter relaxation (LESR). Lower esophageal respiratory pressure (LESP) represents pressure from mean gastric to mean sphincter pressure. LESR is measured both as percent relaxation from LESP to gastric baseline and as residual pressure above gastric baseline at a low point of relaxation. The area and duration of the total relaxation are also measured.

pressure measurement and to have ended once the pressure exceeds the *mean* baseline pressure. An alternative relaxation end (in case of respiratory artifacts) is measured where the pressure exceeds the *highest* point recorded during baseline measurements. The duration of relaxation is the time that elapses between these two points. The percent relaxation is found by first locating the lowest pressure seen during the relaxation phase and obtaining a mean around it for ½ sec. This drop in pressure is calculated as a percent of the full drop from the LES pressure to the gastric pressure. The residual pressure is the difference between the mean lowest pressure during relaxation and gastric pressure. The area of relaxation is calculated as the integral from the relaxation curve to the lower esophageal sphincter pressure.

Analysis of the Upper Esophageal Sphincter

The upper esophageal sphincter (UES) can also be analyzed by both an RPT and an SPT technique, although the analysis of the relaxation phase is much more complex. The computer analysis of UES pressures is analogous to the analysis of LES pressures. Four orifices at the same level oriented radially at 90° are located in the body of the esophagus and pulled through the sphincter. During the pull-through, a high-pressure zone is located. The actual sphincter pressure is reported as the mean of the four high-pressure zones. Sphincter relaxation is measured with three orifices in the sphincter and one in the pharynx. During a swallow there is a pharyngeal contraction closely corresponding to the upper sphincter relaxation. The parameters of interest are those concerned with the timing and coordination of this contraction – relaxation complex and are shown in Figure 7.7. There are six time periods of interest: (1) the time from the beginning of the sphincter relaxation to the beginning of the pharyngeal contraction; (2) the time from the beginning of the sphincter relaxation to the peak of the pharyngeal contraction; (3) the time from the beginning of the sphincter relaxation until the end of the pharyngeal contraction; (4) the duration of the sphincter relaxation; (5) the time from the nadir of the sphincter relaxation to the peak of the pharyngeal contraction; and (6) the time from the beginning of the sphincter relaxation to the end of the sphincter relaxation. The computer program measures a sphincter baseline and defines the beginning of the relaxation as the first time the sphincter pressure falls below the lowest point measured during the baseline period. The nadir of the relaxation is, of course, the lowest sphincter pressure measured during the swallow. The end of the relaxation is defined as the point when the sphincter pressure becomes equal to or greater than the highest pressure recorded during the sphincter baseline measuring period. The beginning of the pharyngeal contraction is defined as the first pressure that exceeds the highest pressure measured

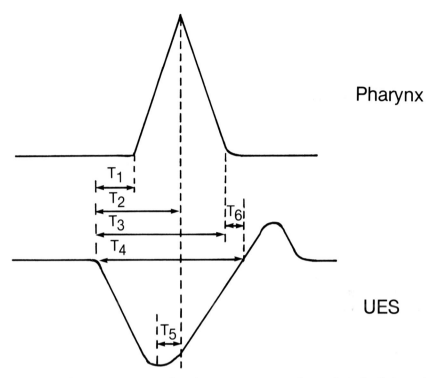

FIGURE 7.7 Schematic representation of parameters measured to evaluate the timing and coordination between upper esophageal sphincter (UES) relaxation and contraction of the pharynx. T_1, time from onset of UES relaxation to onset of pharyngeal contraction; T_2, time from onset of UES relaxation to peak of pharyngeal contraction; T_3, time from onset of UES relaxation to end of pharyngeal contraction; T_4, total duration of UES relaxation; T_5, time from nadir of UES relaxation to peak of pharyngeal contraction; T_6, time from end of pharyngeal contraction to end of UES relaxation.

during the pharyngeal baseline period. The peak of the contraction is the highest pressure measured during the swallow and the end of the contraction is when the pressure is again equal to or less than the highest pressure measured during the pharyngeal baseline sampling. In addition to the timing parameters the program also measures the percent of the sphincter relaxation as compared to baseline, the residual sphincter pressure as compared to the esophageal baseline, and the area of the relaxation measured as the integral from the sphincter baseline to the relaxation curve.

Computer analysis of these three areas allows the investigator a fairly complete pressure profile of the entire esophagus. Interpretations of the studies are consistent and unbiased by expectation. The results are available quickly and data can easily be accumulated for further analysis.

PART II

ABNORMAL ESOPHAGEAL MOTILITY

CHAPTER **8**

Achalasia

Philip O. Katz, MD

Achalasia, or cardiospasm, is the best known and characterized primary esophageal motility disorder. It is a disease of unknown etiology, characterized clinically by slowly progressive dysphagia for solid and liquid food and associated with "obstruction" to esophageal emptying in the absence of an organic legion.

Its pathogenesis resolves around two basic defects: (1) failure of relaxation of a hypertensive or normotensive lower esophageal sphincter (LES) and (2) absent peristalsis in the esophageal body. The diagnosis of achalasia is suggested by a combination of typical clinical and radiologic findings and is confirmed by specific esophageal manometric criteria. This chapter will briefly review the clinical and radiologic findings in achalasia and discuss in detail the manometric findings seen in this disease.

CLINICAL PRESENTATION

Achalasia most commonly presents in the fifth and sixth decades of life, but it may be seen at any age. Males and females present with equal frequency. The classic presentation is longstanding, slowly progressive, painless dysphagia for both solids and liquids. The mean duration of dysphagia is between 5 and 6 years, although it is not unusual to encounter patients with greater than 10 to 20 years of symptoms. The dysphagia is often aggravated by emotional stress. Weight loss is frequent and may be massive. Nocturnal regurgitation may become a prominent manifestation. The disease may thus present with pulmonary symptoms, such as aspiration, wheezing, chronic cough, or choking. Many patients, particularly those with so called "vigorous" achalasia (see below), will have chest pain. Heartburn is not typical, so the symptoms of nocturnal regurgitation and cough in the absence of heartburn should suggest achalasia rather than gastroesophageal (GE) reflux. Rapid onset of symptoms, especially accompanied by rapid, significant weight loss, should suggest achalasia secondary to malignancy.[1]

RADIOLOGIC FEATURES

The diagnosis of achalasia may be suggested on plain chest x-ray with the findings of a widened mediastinum — from a dilated esophagus — and the absence of a gastric air bubble. Barium esophagram will reveal a dilated esophagus, often with a midesophageal air-fluid level, and smooth distal tapering in a "bird-breaking" configuration (cardiospasm). Fluoroscopy will demonstrate the absence of esophageal peristalsis and delayed emptying of barium. The presence of smooth distal tapering helps differentiate achalasia from the more shaggy, ragged appearance of a distal esophageal carcinoma or a peptic stricture. The air-fluid level and "tight" gastroesophageal junction help separate achalasia from scleroderma, in which barium is retained in the supine position but empties rapidly when the patient is upright (hence no fluid level). The gastroesophageal junction in scleroderma is also usually wide open.

Radionuclide transit studies, in which a gamma camera is used to follow a bolus of a radiolabeled liquid or solid meal down the esophagus, have proved useful in evaluating patients with suspected achalasia. Liquid-emptying studies show an adynamic pattern of emptying and delayed emptying in the upright position.[2] Solid-meal emptying in the upright position can give useful information about sphincter function and is particularly helpful in atypical cases (see below) as well as in assessing response to therapy.[3]

ENDOSCOPY

Though useful in the diagnosis of many upper gastrointestinal diseases, the value of the endoscopy in achalasia is mainly one of exclusion. All patients with suspected achalasia should undergo endoscopy to rule out carcinoma simulating achalasia and to rule out short peptic strictures. Typical, but not diagnostic, endoscopic features of achalasia include a patulous esophageal body with a tight LES that will not open with air insufflation, but opens relatively easily with gentle pressure of the endoscope against the GE junction. A retroflexed view of the gastroesophageal junction is essential to help exclude occult malignancy.

MANOMETRY

The above features will strongly suggest a diagnosis of achalasia. The diagnosis should always be confirmed by esophageal manometry. Four manometric findings are characteristic of achalasia: (1) absence of peristalsis in the esophageal body, (2) incomplete or abnormal LES relaxation, (3) elevated LES pressure, and (4) elevated intraesophageal pressures relative to the gastric baseline. Absent peristalsis is an absolute requirement for diagnosis. Incomplete LES relaxation is usually seen but may be absent, particularly when manometry is performed in early achalasia. As a group, patients with achalasia have LES pressures greater than normal but overlap does exist,[4] so a normal LES pressure does not rule out this diagnosis. Elevated esophageal pressures relative to gastric pressure are seen but are not required (Table 8.1).

Several technical problems may occur in the performance of manometry in patients with suspected achalasia. Though the technical aspects of performing a manometric exam have been discussed in Chapter 4, several points pertinent to achalasia should be made. These patients often have an extremely dilated, tortuous esophagus, and difficulty may therefore be encountered in passing the catheter, due to curling in the esophageal body. Remember that these patients have difficulty swallowing, so large amounts of liquids should not be given to "help pass the tube." Failure of the LES to open may preclude passage of the catheter into the stomach. The operator should be gentle, and attempt to pass the tube slowly. Fluoroscopy is occasionally needed to confirm the location of the tube and aid in passage into the stomach. The inability to obtain a gastric baseline pattern is a clue that the catheter is still in the esophagus and should alert the examiner to the possibility of achalasia.

LOWER ESOPHAGEAL SPHINCTER

If the catheter can be passed into the stomach, it is usually preferable to perform the station pull-through (SPT) technique of LES measurement

TABLE 8.1 Manometric Findings in Achalasia

Absent peristalsis in esophageal body (required for diagnosis)
Incomplete lower esophageal sphincter relaxation (usually present, not required); short duration relaxation may be only finding in early achalasia
Hypertensive lower sphincter (common, not required)
Elevated intraesophageal pressures relative to gastric pressure (occasional, not required)

immediately, rather than a rapid pull-through (RPT) as is suggested for most exams. The SPT allows assessment of both LES pressure and LES relaxation, which cannot be done with the RPT technique.

LES relaxation should be assessed with wet swallows (5 mL), since dry swallows may cause underestimation of relaxation[5] and give the false impression of incomplete relaxation in normal individuals. It is our practice to give at least one wet swallow per station at the point when the catheter is positioned in the maximum high-pressure zone of the LES. A total of at least six swallows should be measured during a study to permit adequate assessment of LES relaxation. Relaxation should be considered normal if LES pressure drops greater than 90% from mean resting LES pressure to gastric baseline (GBL) pressure.[6] Most patients with achalasia will have obvious incomplete relaxation, with measurement of the actual percentage being unimportant (Fig. 8.1). It is important to be aware that patients with early achalasia may have apparently complete LES relaxation on the manometry tracing (see below).[4]

In addition to recording LES relaxation as the percent drop in pressure to gastric pressure, it is often helpful to evaluate the duration of LES relaxation, an assessment of the time the sphincter is actually open. Though little attention has been paid to duration of relaxation in the literature, we have found this measurement particularly useful for patients in whom achalasia is suspected, but who demonstrate apparently complete LES percent relaxation. Many of these patients will demonstrate a shorter duration of relaxation compared to normals (Fig. 8.2). A recent series reported seven patients with clinical and radiologic characteristics of achalasia, in whom manometry demonstrated absent peristalsis but normal LES percent relaxation.[4] A short duration of LES relaxation was the only sphincter abnormality noted in this group (Table 8.2). In our laboratory, assessment of relaxation duration can aid in the manometric diagnosis of achalasia.

In addition to finding complete and short duration LES relaxation, it is quite common to find a hypertensive LES (Fig. 8.3). Pressures may be so high that it is necessary for the examiner to readjust the gain on the recorder to interpret LES pressure accurately. If this is done, a new GBL must be obtained to accurately measure pressure and assess relaxation.

ESOPHAGEAL BODY

Elevated esophageal pressures relative to the GBL are occasionally seen in patients with achalasia (Fig. 8.4). If this is the case, the examiner will fail to see the normal pressure drop to below GBL as the catheter moves out of the sphincter into the esophageal body. In this case, it is important to confirm

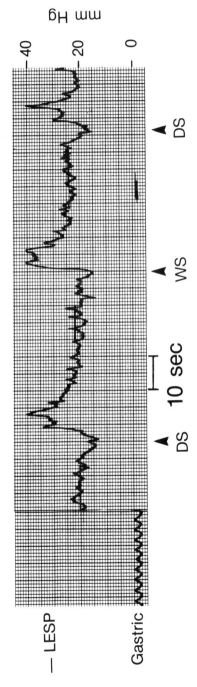

FIGURE 8.1 Incomplete LES relaxation after both wet (WS) and dry (DS) swallows in a patient with achalasia. Note that mean LES pressure (LESP) (23 mm Hg) falls within the normal range for our laboratory.

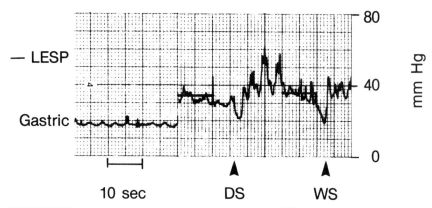

FIGURE 8.2 Patient with early achalasia who has incomplete LES relaxation with dry swallows (DS) but complete relaxation to GBL baseline with wet swallows (WS). The duration of relaxation, measured from the initial decline to the return of the resting LES pressure (LESP) is shortened (approximately 4 sec).

that the catheter is indeed in the body by the characteristic drop in pressure with respiration.

Motility in the esophageal body is assessed with wet swallows. Patients with achalasia will demonstrate total absence of primary peristalsis, ie, simultaneous contractions of the entire smooth muscle of the body in response to a water swallow (Fig. 8.5). Contractions are usually of low amplitude, (20–40 mm Hg) and may be difficult to distinguish from respiratory artifact. When the esophagus is extremely dilated, no contractions will be seen in response to a swallow.

ATYPICAL FINDINGS

There is a subgroup of patients, with complete absence of peristalsis, and the other manometric features of achalasia, who exhibit higher-amplitude

TABLE 8.2 Duration of Lower Esophageal Sphincter Relaxation in Achalasia and Normal Subjects

	Duration (sec; $\bar{x} \pm$ SE)	P Value
Normals (N = 20)	11.7 ± 0.6	<0.01
Early achalasia (N = 7)[a]	7.2 ± 0.6	
Long-standing achalasia (N = 16)	7.1 ± 0.6	NS[b]

[a]Achalasia patients with apparent complete percent relaxation.
[b]NS, not significant.

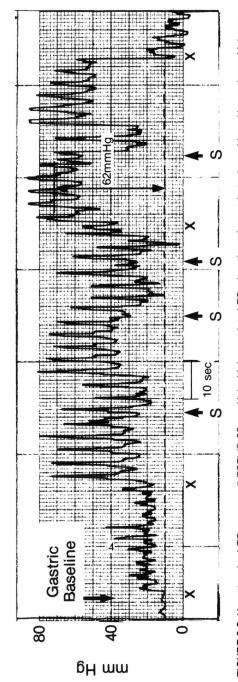

FIGURE 8.3 Hypertensive LES pressure (LESP) ($\bar{x}$: 62 mm Hg) with incomplete LES relaxation when catheter is positioned in maximum high-pressure zone of the sphincter. x, tube moved up 0.5 cm; S, swallow.

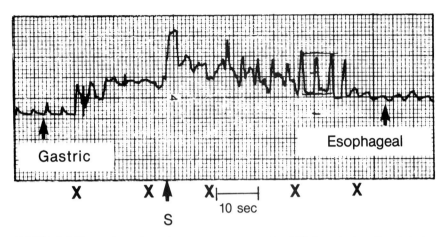

X   X↑   X├────┤   X   X
              S   10 sec

FIGURE 8.4 Elevated esophageal pressures compared to GBL in patients with achalasia. Increased baseline esophageal pressures are usually the result of retained fluids in a relatively closed system. x, tube moved up 0.5 cm; S, swallow.

(greater than 60 mm Hg) simultaneous repetitive contractions in response to swallows (Fig. 8.6). This manometric pattern is called *vigorous* achalasia.[7,8] This group is differentiated from patients with more *classic* achalasia, in that they have a greater incidence of severe chest pain and less esophageal dilation on x-ray.[7] LES relaxation is usually incomplete and peristalsis is absent, as in patients with more typical manometric findings of achalasia.

Another subgroup of patients, with all the clinical and radiologic hallmarks of achalasia, have manometry that demonstrates apparently normal LES relaxation and absence of peristalsis in the esosphageal body. In a recently reported series, 30% of all patients seen with achalasia in a 2-year period demonstrated these manometric findings.[4] Another study of 135 patients with aperistalsis found that 19% had normal LES relaxation[8] suggesting that this manometric combination is quite common. These patients usually present with clinical and radiologic findings suggestive of achalasia, although they typically have shorter duration of dysphagia and less weight loss than those with longstanding disease. Barium esophagrams will demonstrate absent peristalsis and the smooth "bird-beak" tapering, but less dilatation than patients with longer duration of disease. Esophageal manometry demonstrates relaxation of the LES to the GBL, but a significantly shorter duration of relaxation than in normals. The esophageal body demonstrates complete aperistalsis. This group represents an early stage of true achalasia and not a nonspecific motility disorder. If the diagnosis is still in doubt, an upright radionuclide solid-emptying study should be done to confirm abnormal emptying.[4]

TREATMENT

A detailed discussion of treatment is beyond the scope of this chapter. Key points in treatment and their effect on the manometric findings will be briefly discussed.

The aim of therapy is to reduce LES pressure and allow esophageal emptying, while retaining enough residual pressure to prevent GE reflux. This can be done equally well by pneumatic dilatation or esophageal myo-

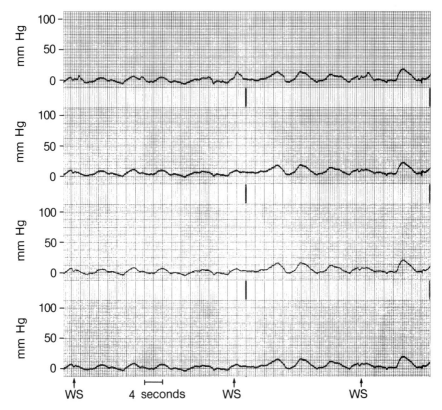

FIGURE 8.5 Total absence of peristalsis in the esophageal body. All contractions are simultaneous, and low amplitude, and may be difficult to distinguish from respiratory artifact. WS, wet swallow.

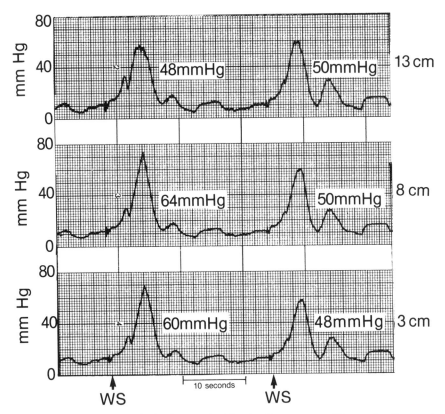

FIGURE 8.6 Vigorous achalasia characterized by simultaneous, repetitive contractions and with higher amplitude than observed in the classic form of achalasia. WS, wet swallow.

tomy, although a higher likelihood of reflux may accompany myotomy.[9] Each procedure gives good to excellent results with minimal complications when properly performed. Pneumatic dilatation should be performed as the primary therapy, with surgery reserved for those who do not respond. Therapy with calcium-channel blockers,[10] nitrates,[10] and, occasionally, mercury bougie dilatation has demonstrated symptomatic improvement in some series, but should be reserved for patients with early disease, minimal dysphagia, and little esophageal dilation.

Repeat esophageal manometry is usually not necessary as a follow up to treatment, provided that symptoms improve. If medical therapy is attempted, radionuclide studies may be useful to evaluate improvement in emptying.[3] Several manometric changes may be seen if follow-up manometry is done. LES pressure will decrease and may be low, predisposing the patient to reflux. In most cases LES relaxation will remain incomplete but it is not unusual to see some complete relaxations in response to wet swallows. Somewhat more controversial is the question of return of peristalsis. Under most circumstances no peristalsis returns. However a few case reports[11,12] have demonstrated return of peristalsis after treatment. Vantrappen and colleagues[8] found some normal peristaltic sequence in 22 of 69 patients with aperistalsis, who were treated with pneumatic dilitation, so it seems that on rare occasions some peristalsis may be seen if manometry is performed after treatment.

REFERENCES

1. Tucker JH, Snape WJ, Cohen S: Achalasia secondary to carcinoma. Manometric and clinical features. *Ann Intern Med* 1978;89:315.
2. Russell COH, Hill LD, Holmes ER III, et al: Radionuclide transit: A sensitive screening test for esophageal dysfunction. *Gastroenterology*, 1981;80:887–892.
3. Holloway RH, Krisin G, Lange RC, et al: Radionuclide esophageal emptying of a solid meal and quantitative results of therapy in achalasia. *Gastroenterology* 1983;84:771–776.
4. Katz PO, Richter JE, Cowan R, et al: Apparent complete lower esophageal sphincter relaxation in achalasia. *Gastroenterology* 1986;90:978–983.
5. Chobanian SJ, Benjamin SB, Spurling TJ, et al: Characterization of lower esophageal sphincter relaxation in normals (abstr). *Clin Res* 1982;80:723A.
6. Cohen S, Lipschultz W: Lower esophageal sphincter dysfunction in achalasia. *Gastroenterology* 1971;61:814–820.
7. Bondi JL, Godwin DH, Garrett JM: "Vigorous" achalasia: it's clinical interpretation and significance. *Am J Gastroenterol* 1972;58:145–154.
8. Vantrappen G, Janssens J, Hellemans J, et al: Achalasia, diffuse esophageal spasm and related motility disorders. *Gastroenterology* 1979;76:450–457.
9. Vantrappen G, Hellemans J: Treatment of achalasia and related motor disorders. *Gastroenterology* 1980;79:144–154.
10. Gelfand M, Rosen P, Keren S, et al: Isosorbide dinitrate and nifedipine treatment of achalasia: A clinical, manometric and radionuclide evaluation. *Gastroenterology* 1982;83:963–969.
11. Mellow MH: Return of esophageal peristalsis in idiopathic achalasia. *Gastroenterology* 1976;70:1148–1151.
12. Bianco A, Cagossi M, Scrimieri D, et al: Appearance of esophageal peristalsis in treated idiopathic achalasia. *Dig Dis Sci* 1986;31:40–48.

CHAPTER 9

Diffuse Esophageal Spasm

Joel E. Richter, MD, FACP

Diffuse esophageal spasm is a clinical syndrome characterized by symptoms of substernal chest pain and/or dysphagia, tertiary contractions on x-ray, and a manometric pattern characterized by frequent simultaneous contractions mixed with normal peristalsis. The areas of ignorance and controversy concerning this disorder are great. Recent improvements in manometric techniques, and a better understanding of the variations in normal esophageal motility, now permit a better definition of diffuse esophageal spasm.

HISTORICAL BACKGROUND

The clinical syndrome of diffuse esophageal spasm was first described by Hamilton Osgood in 1889.[1] His descriptive monograph on six patients with esophageal chest pain is still remarkably accurate, even to the characteristic relief of symptoms by "nitrate of silver" (nitroglycerin). The earliest manometric studies of diffuse esophageal spasm were done by Creamer and associates[2] and Roth and Fleshler[3] and published in 1958 and 1964, respectively. Using a highly compliant manometric system and dry swallows, these investigators identified the manometric feature common to patients with diffuse spasm: the simultaneous onset or peak of pressure contractions recorded by two adjacent recording orifices in the esophagus. The simultaneous waves, usually in the distal esophagus, were mixed with normal peristaltic sequences, showing that the esophagus had not completely lost its ability to produce peristaltic contractions, thereby suggesting a partial or intermittent defect. Other reported manometric abnormalities, although less consistent, included repetitive waves, high contraction pressures, and prolonged duration of contractions. These latter findings were usually not seen as isolated events, but occurred as variations of the basic abnormal response, ie, simultaneous contractions.

As shown in Table 9.1, subsequent authors have attempted to refine the manometric criteria for diffuse esophageal spasm. In doing so, these reports may have de-emphasized the importance of the simultaneous contraction. In fact, so much attention has been given to diffuse esophageal spasm as the "classic" esophageal motility disorder that this diagnosis has become misused as a catchall term for patients with noncardiac chest pain.[15] Recent series, however, suggest that diffuse esophageal spasm may account for only 5% to 15% of the esophageal motility disorders identified in noncardiac chest-pain patients.[16,17]

PATHOPHYSIOLOGY AND ETIOLOGY

As is true with many esophageal motility disorders, the etiology and pathophysiology of diffuse esophageal spasm are not known. Pathologic information is sparse because this syndrome rarely leads to death or even to an operation during which tissue may be obtained. The most striking pathologic change reported grossly in the esophagus has been diffuse muscular thickening, mainly of the lower two-thirds of the esophagus.[5,18] There are other well-documented cases of diffuse esophageal spasm in which muscular thickening was not found at thoracotomy.[19] Unlike achalasia, ganglion cells are not reduced in number. One report did find diffuse changes in the vagus nerve, characterized by fragmentation of neural filaments, increase in endoneural collagen, and fragmentation of mitochondria.[5]

SYMPTOMS

Chest pain and dysphagia are the main clinical complaints. These symptoms are intermittent, and vary from mild and occasional to severe and daily. The chest pain is located substernally and may radiate directly through to the back and shoulder blades. The pain is not necessarily related to the act of swallowing. However, it can sometimes be triggered by the ingestion of either very hot or very cold liquids. It frequently awakes the patient from sleep and may worsen during periods of emotional stress. The pain may closely mimic angina pectoris, even to the point of being relieved by nitroglycerin. The dysphagia is of variable severity and lacks the persistence seen in achalasia or organic stenosis. It does not necessarily accompany chest pain and occurs

TABLE 9.1 Summary of Previously Published Manometric Criteria for Diffuse Esophageal Spasm

Year	Reference	Intermittent Peristalsis	Simultaneous Contractions	Repetitive	Spontaneous	High Amplitude	Prolonged Duration	Abnormal LES
1958	Creamer et al[2]	–	+	+ (> 1 peak)	–	+	+	–
1964	Roth and Fleshler[3]	+	+	+	–	–	+	–
1966	Craddock et al[4]	–	+	+	–	+	–	–
1967	Gillies et al[5]	–	+	+ (2–5 peaks)	+	–	+ (> 6 sec)	–
1970	Bennett and Hendrix[6]	–	+	+	+	+	–	–
1973	Orlando and Bozymski[7]	–	+	+	+	+	–	+
1974	DiMarino and Cohen[8]	+	+ (> 30%)	+	–	+	–	+ (1/3)
1977	Mellow[9]	+	+ (> 30%)	+	–	+ (> 35 mm Hg)	+ (> 7.5 sec)	–
1977	Swamy[10]	–	+	+	+	+	–	–
1979	Vantrappen et al[11]	+	+	+ (≥ 3 peaks)	–	+ (> 70 mm Hg)	+ (> 6 sec)	+
1981	Kaye[12]	+	+	+	–	+	+	+ (2/3)
1982	Davies et al[13]	+	+ (> 10%)	+	+	+ (> 50 mm Hg)	+ (> 12 sec)	+
1982	Patterson[14]	+	+	–	–	+ (> 120 mm Hg)	–	–

after the ingestion of both liquids and solids. Food impaction,[2] syncope on swallowing,[3] and weight loss from fear of eating[5] have been described, but are unusual clinical features of diffuse esophageal spasm.

MANOMETRIC DIAGNOSIS

Any meaningful current manometric definition of diffuse esophageal spasm must take into consideration the recent advances in instrumentation and methodology used to evaluate esophageal motor function. Low-compliance pneumohydraulic infusion pumps or miniature intraesophageal pressure transducers now allow accurate pressure measurements from the esophageal body as well as the lower esophageal sphincter (LES). Before the newer technology, a contraction pressure of more than 40 to 50 mm Hg was considered one of high amplitude.[20] Wet swallows of water have now replaced dry swallows as the conventional means to induce peristaltic activity. Among healthy subjects, simultaneous contractions may follow 15% to 30% of dry swallows, but are rare after wet swallows (see Chapter 6). These improvements, combined with a better understanding of the variations of normal esophageal activity,[16,21] now allow us to more precisely define the manometric criteria for diffuse esophageal spasm (Table 9.2).

Simultaneous Contractions

The presence of frequent simultaneous contractions after wet swallows, mixed with normal peristalsis, are the sine qua non for the manometric diagnosis of diffuse esophageal spasm. This is the one manometric abnormality that has been consistently described in all reports on diffuse esophageal spasm (Table 9.1). We believe all other reported manometric abnormal-

TABLE 9.2 Manometric Criteria for Diffuse Esophageal Spasm

Required
    Simultaneous contractions ($>$ 10% of wet swallows)
    Intermittent normal peristalsis
Associated findings
    Repetitive contractions ($\geq$ 3 peaks)
    Prolonged duration of contractions
    High-amplitude contractions
    Frequent spontaneous contractions
    Lower esophageal sphincter abnormalities
        Incomplete relaxation
        High resting pressures

ities are associated findings that, by themselves, do not constitute diffuse esophageal spasm.[15] Based on our experience with 95 healthy adults, simultaneous contractions are uncommon after wet swallows, ie, four subjects who each had only one simultaneous contraction in a series of ten wet swallows. Therefore, we define diffuse esophageal spasm by the presence of greater than 10% simultaneous contractions. In a recent review of 40 patients with symptomatic diffuse esophageal spasm, we observed simultaneous contractions after approximately 40% of wet swallows (range 20%–90%) (Fig. 9.1). A minimum of 30% simultaneous contractions has been proposed for the diagnostic criterion of diffuse esophageal spasm when using dry swallows.[8,9] However, we do not believe dry swallows should be used to

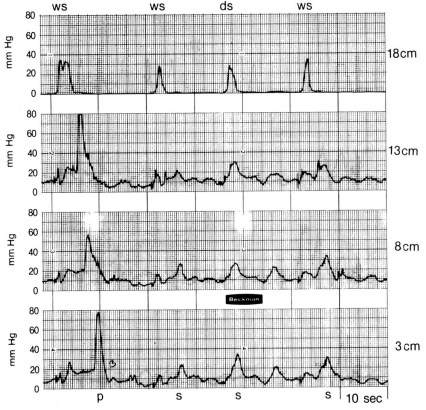

FIGURE 9.1 Frequent simultaneous contractions (s) after wet swallows (ws) intermixed with normal peristaltic activity (p) in a patient with diffuse esophageal spasm. Note the relatively low amplitude and normal duration of the simultaneous contractions. ds, dry swallow.

diagnose esophageal motility disorders, because simultaneous contractions may be seen after 80% and even 100% of dry swallows in healthy adults (Fig.9.2).

The mere presence of simultaneous contractions is not sufficient for a diagnosis of diffuse esophageal spasm. Simultaneous contractions can be seen in patients with gastroesophageal (GE) reflux,[10,22] neuropathies secondary to diabetes, collagen vascular diseases, pseudo-obstruction, and alcoholism.[23,24] These patients can usually be distinguished by history or physical examination. The simultaneous contractions associated with neuropathies are also generally asymptomatic. If all pressure waves are simultaneous, a diagnosis of achalasia must be entertained even if the LES appears to relax.[25]

Repetitive Contractions

Repetitive waves are commonly reported in diffuse esophageal spasm (Table 9.1) but the criterion for the number of abnormal peaks has varied among series. Earlier investigators[2,5] defined repetitive contractions as two or more pressure peaks in response to a single swallow, while more recent studies require the presence of at least three peaks.[11,16] In our laboratory, double-peaked waves are relatively common in healthy adults, occurring after 11% to 18% of swallows (see Chapter 6). Triple-peaked waves are rare, occurring after 0.1% of wet swallows (one triple-peaked wave in 950 wet swallows). Therefore, triple-peaked waves, but not double-peaked waves, are an indication of disordered esophageal motility. We observed repetitive contractions ($\geq$ 3 peaks) in 12 out of 40 (30%) patients with diffuse esophageal spasm. In these patients, the frequency of repetitive contractions ranged from 10% to 40% (Fig. 9.3). Repetitive contractions may be swallow induced or spontaneous (not related to a swallow). We do not make a diagnosis of diffuse esophageal spasm when triple-peaked waves are not associated with the presence of simultaneous contractions.

Contractions of High Amplitude and Prolonged Duration

Giant contraction waves have long been recognized as occurring frequently with diffuse esophageal spasm.[2] It has traditionally been thought that these giant simultaneous contractions are the cause of a patient's chest pain and dysphagia. Mellow has proposed that a mean esophageal contraction duration of greater than 7.5 sec should suggest diffuse esophageal spasm.[9] The significance of high-amplitude contractions in the diagnosis of diffuse esophageal spasm has been called into question because the older, less accurate high-compliance systems used in older studies *underestimate* the pressures normally generated in the body of the esophagus. In our experience, mean

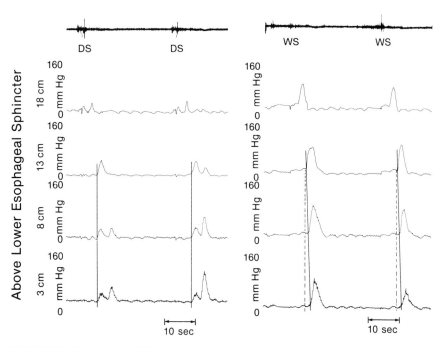

FIGURE 9.2 Dry swallows (DS) may cause overestimation of the frequency of simultaneous contractions. As demonstrated in this healthy volunteer, all dry swallows are followed by simultaneous distal contraction. In contrast, all wet swallows (WS) are followed by orderly peristaltic contractions. Wet swallows should always be used to assess simultaneous activity.

esophageal pressures of high amplitude and prolonged duration are uncommon in diffuse esophageal spasm and are only associated findings in the manometric diagnosis. In 40 patients with diffuse esophageal spasm, diagnosed in our laboratory over the last 4 years, the mean distal contraction amplitude was 84 mm Hg (range 41–216 mm Hg), with individual contractions ranging from 16–350 mm Hg. Likewise, mean distal contraction duration usually was within the normal range for our laboratory (<6.0 sec), with a mean duration of 3.8 sec (range 3.0–7.0 sec) and individual contractions ranging from 3.0–12.0 sec (Fig. 9.4). If all pressure waves are peristaltic, but of high amplitude and prolonged duration, a diagnosis of nutcracker esophagus rather than diffuse esophageal spasm should be made.

Frequent Spontaneous Contractions

Gillies and associates[5] were the first to report frequent spontaneous contractions associated with simultaneous and repetitive activity, but this has not been a common criteria for diffuse esophageal spasm in other reports (Table 9.1). We have found that 50% of healthy adults will have spontaneous esophageal activity when studied manometrically during a 5-min quiet period. The frequency of these "normal" spontaneous contractions ranges from one per 5-min period to many simultaneous, repetitive contractions that resemble diffuse esophageal spasm (Fig. 9.5). This observation suggests that frequent spontaneous activity may be a variation of the normal and must be interpreted cautiously in the diagnosis of diffuse esophageal spasm.

Lower Esophageal Sphincter Abnormalities

Most patients with diffuse esophageal spasm have normal lower esophageal sphincter (LES) pressures and complete sphincter relaxation upon swal-

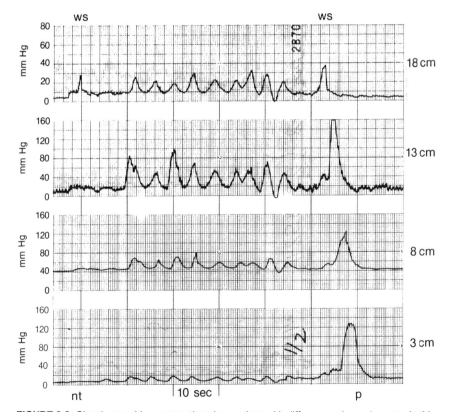

FIGURE 9.3 Classic repetitive contractions in a patient with diffuse esophageal spasm. In this case, the nontransmitted (nt) wet swallow (ws) resulted in pooling of fluid in the body of the esophagus and subsequent repetitive, simultaneous contractions. This is terminated by a peristaltic contraction (p) after a wet swallow.

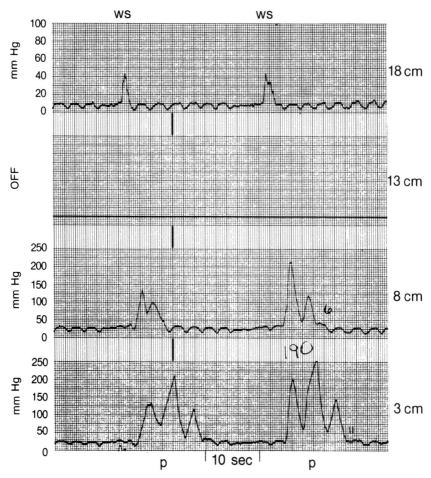

FIGURE 9.4 A segment of a motility tracing from a patient with diffuse esophageal spasm (30% of the contractions were simultaneous). Two wet swallows (ws) are followed by peristaltic contractions (p), which have triple-peaked, high-amplitude, prolonged duration contractions at the most distal recording site.

lowing. DiMarino and Cohen[8] reported that LES relaxation was incomplete in 10 patients and hypertensive sphincters were found in 9 of 27 patients with diffuse esophageal spasm. Incomplete sphincter relaxation occurred even more frequently (8 out of 12 patients) in another series of patients with diffuse esophageal spasm.[12] In our review of 40 patients with diffuse spasm, we also observed incomplete LES relaxation in two patients and a third patient had a hypertensive sphincter. Whether the finding of "complete" relaxation by manometry means that the sphincter opens normally or merely indicates that it has relaxed to the point where its minimal diameter is as great as that of the recording catheter is an interesting point.[12] Recent studies in patients with early achalasia suggest that "apparent" complete LES relaxation may be an artifact of our measurement techniques, since it is associated with abnormal upright esophageal emptying of a solid meal.[25] These abnormalities in LES function, combined with follow-up studies confirming the evolution of diffuse esophageal spasm to achalasia, strongly

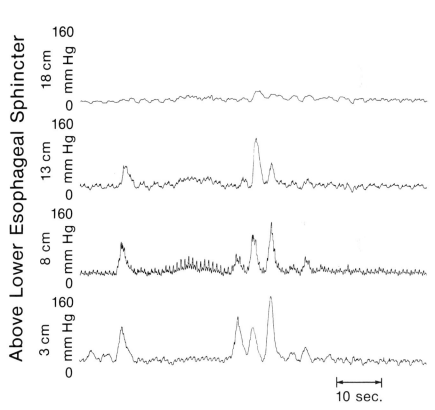

FIGURE 9.5 Frequent spontaneous contractions either isolated or associated with simultaneous, repetitive activity may be seen in diffuse esophageal spasm. However, healthy volunteers may have similar activity and this manometric feature must be interpreted cautiously in the diagnosis of diffuse esophageal spasm. Note that the recording at the top shows no evidence of swallow activity.

suggest these disorders may represent a dynamic spectrum of esophageal motility dysfunction.[11,26]

CONCLUSIONS

Diffuse esophageal spasm does not have to be a confusing, vague syndrome. Detailed investigations into the normal variations of esophageal contraction pressures currently permit a more precise manometric definition of this motility disorder. Overall, our experience does little more than re-emphasize the basic criteria for diffuse esophageal spasm suggested by earlier investigators, ie, simultaneous contractions mixed with normal peristalsis. Diffuse esophageal spasm, however, is an uncommon motility disorder and should not be used as a generic term to describe patients with suspected esophageal chest pains.

REFERENCES

1. Osgood H: A peculiar form of oesophagismus. *Boston Medical and Surgical Journal* 1889;120:401–405.
2. Creamer B, Donoghue FE, Code CF: Pattern of esophageal motility in diffuse spasm. *Gastroenterology* 1958;34:782–796.
3. Roth HP, Fleshler B: Diffuse esophageal spasm. *Ann Intern Med* 1964;61:914–923.
4. Craddock DR, Logan A, Walabaum PR: Diffuse esophageal spasm. *Thorax* 1966;21:511–517.
5. Gillies M, Nicks R, Skyring A: Clinical, manometric, and pathological studies in diffuse oesophageal spasm. *Br Med J* 1967;2:527–530.
6. Bennett JR, Hendrix TR: Diffuse esophageal spasm: a disorder with more than one cause. *Gastroenterology* 1970;59:273–279.
7. Orlando RC, Bozymski EM: Clinical and manometric effects of nitroglycerin in diffuse esophageal spasm. *N Engl J Med* 1973;289:23–25.
8. DiMarino AJ, Cohen S: Characteristics of lower esophageal sphincter function in symptomatic diffuse esophageal spasm. *Gastroenterology* 1974;66:1–6.
9. Mellow M: Symptomatic diffuse esophageal spasm: manometric follow-up and response to cholinergic stimulation and cholinesterase inhibition. *Gastroenterology* 1977;73:237–240.
10. Swamy N: Esophageal spasm and manometric response to nitroglycerin and long acting nitrates. *Gastroenterology* 1977;72:23–27.
11. Vantrappen G, Janssens J, Hellerman J, et al: Achalasia, diffuse esophageal spasm, and related motility disorders. *Gastroenterology* 1979;76:450–457.
12. Kaye MD: Anomalies of peristalsis in idiopathic diffuse oesophageal spasm. *Gut* 1981;22:217–222.
13. Alban-Davies H, Kay MD, Rhodes J, et al: Diagnosis of oesophageal spasm by ergometrine provocation. *Gut* 1982;23:89–97.
14. Patterson DR: Diffuse esophageal spasm in patients with undiagnosed chest pain. *J Clin Gastroenterol* 1982;4:415–417.

15. Richter JE, Castell DO: Diffuse esophageal spasm: a reappraisal. *Ann Intern Med* 1984;100:242–245.
16. Clouse RE, Staiano A: Contraction abnormalities of the esophageal body in patients referred for manometry: a new approach to manometric classification. *Dig Dis Sci* 1983;28:784–791.
17. Katz PO, Dalton CB, Richter JE, et al: Esophageal testing of patients with non-cardiac chest pain and/or dysphagia. Results of a three year experience with 1161 patients. *Ann Intern Med* 1987;106:593–597.
18. Ferguson TB, Woodbury JD, Roper CL: Giant muscular hypertrophy of the esophagus. *Ann Thorac Surg* 1969;8:209–212.
19. Ellis FH, Olsen AM, Schlegal JF, et al: Surgical treatment of esophageal hypermotility disturbances. *JAMA* 1964;188:862–866.
20. Nagler R, Spiro HM: Serial esophageal motility studies in asymptomatic young subjects. *Gastroenterology* 1961,41:371–379.
21. Richter JE, Wu WC, Johns DN, et al: Esophageal manometry in 95 healthy adult volunteers: variability of pressure with age and frequency of "abnormal" contractions. *Dig Dis Sci* (in press).
22. Ahtaridis A, Snape WJ, Cohen S: Clinical and manometric findings in benign peptic strictures of the esophagus. *Dig Dis Sci* 1979;24:858–861.
23. Winship DH, Caflisch CR, Aboralske FF, et al: Deterioration of esophageal peristalsis in patients with alcoholic neuropathy. *Gastroenterology* 1968;55:173–178.
24. Hollis, JB, Castell DO, Braddon RL: Esophageal function in diabetes mellitus and its relation to peripheral neuropathy. *Gastroenterology* 1977;73:1098–1102.
25. Katz PO, Richter JE, Cowan R, et al: Apparent complete lower esophageal sphincter relaxation in achalasia. *Gastroenterology* 1986;90:978–983.
26. Castell DO: The spectrum of esophageal motility disorders. *Gastroenterology* 1979;76:639–645.

CHAPTER 10

The Nutcracker Esophagus and Other Primary Esophageal Motility Disorders

Donald O. Castell, MD, FACP

Since the mid 1970s, a remarkable change has occurred in the types of patients being evaluated in esophageal motility laboratories. This is due to the increasing recognition that patients with noncardiac chest pain may frequently demonstrate abnormalities in esophageal contractions. This concept will be discussed more completely in Chapter 11. Prior to the recognition of this phenomenon and the increased utilization of esophageal motility testing in this group of patients, most patients evaluated in motility laboratories presented with either dysphagia or some form of reflux disease. Therefore, the diagnoses usually being sought were either the more traditional primary motility disorders of achalasia or diffuse esophageal spasm, or evidence of a significantly diminished lower esophageal sphincter (LES) pressure.

As increasing numbers of patients with undiagnosed chest pain were evaluated in esophageal motility laboratories, it became clear that other contraction abnormalities in the peristaltic sequence were being seen with greater frequency. Although the traditional concept had been that the esophageal motility abnormality most likely to produce chest pain was diffuse spasm, recent observations have proven that this is not the case. Rather, some new potential primary motility disorders have been described and attempts have been made to classify or categorize some of these contraction abnormalities. In this chapter, an attempt will be made to clarify our concepts of these other primary motility disorders and to describe their presentation.

130

NUTCRACKER ESOPHAGUS

Although the term "nutcracker esophagus" was coined by investigators working in our laboratory, it was never intended to imply any knowledge of the pathophysiology of this common motility finding. Rather, our goal was to use a title that was so unusual that it would create an awareness of the commonplace nature of this entity. Review of the literature over the past few years would seem to indicate that our purpose has been met, for there is now widespread use of the term nutcracker esophagus when describing the patients that have this esophageal motility pattern. Actually, the initial description of high-amplitude peristaltic contractions was first made from the laboratory of Charles Pope in a publication by Brand et al, in which 41% of patients with chest pain and esophageal abnormalities were shown to have excessively large peristaltic waves.[1] Pope has subsequently used the term "super-squeezer" when referring to this group of patients. In 1979, Benjamin et al reported on a similar group of patients who exhibited excessive amplitude of peristaltic contractions. We observed these during our early studies on the increasing numbers of patients with noncardiac chest pain.[2] Other terms that have been used to describe these patients include "hypertensive peristalsis," "symptomatic esophageal peristalsis," and "high-amplitude peristaltic contractions."

By definition, the nutcracker esophagus is a manometric abnormality characterized by an average distal esophageal peristaltic pressure greater than 2 SD above a well-documented normal range in a patient with chest pain and/or dysphagia. In our laboratory, this is defined by average peristaltic pressures (mean of 10 wet swallows) exceeding 180 mm Hg (Fig. 10.1A). We have seen some patients with average unstimulated pressures in excess of 400 mm Hg. These extremely strong peristaltic waves can be shown to respond appropriately to pharmacologic agents that attenuate esophageal contractions, such as atropine (Fig. 10.1B) and nifedipine (Fig. 10.1C). Patients with this manometric diagnosis have been frequently reported in many areas of this country, including Seattle,[1] Oklahoma City,[3] Bethesda,[4] New Haven,[5] New Orleans,[6] and Winston-Salem.[7] The nutcracker esophagus occurs in 27% to 48% of the patients with abnormal esophageal motility described in these reports (summarized in Table 10.1). One additional aspect of the motility abnormality seen in patients with the nutcracker esophagus was described by Herrington et al.[6] In this report, the authors identified a group of patients whose manometric abnormality consisted primarily of excessively long-duration peristaltic waves. In our laboratory, these patients are identified by high-amplitude contractions, although many will also show average durations in excess of 6 sec (Fig. 10.2). Therefore, it is appropriate that prolonged duration peristaltic contractions should be considered part of the spectrum of the nutcracker esophagus.

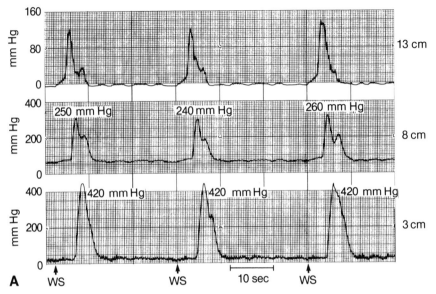

FIGURE 10.1 (A) Motility tracing demonstrating a typical peristaltic response in a patient with a nutcracker esophagus. The three recording sites are located 13, 8, and 3 cm above the LES. The response to three wet swallows (WS) is shown. **(B)** Response to atropine in the same patient demonstrating the marked inhibition of the contraction pressures. **(C)** Response to nifedipine (30 mg orally) demonstrating the marked reduction in peristaltic contractions.

tion peristaltic contractions should be considered part of the spectrum of the nutcracker esophagus.

How is the Nutcracker Esophagus Defined?

As noted above, the manometric diagnosis of the nutcracker esophagus was the direct result of many manometry laboratories experiencing increasing numbers of patients evaluated for unexplained chest pain. In almost every instance, laboratories from all parts of this country were recognizing that a high percentage of these patients had excessively large peristaltic contractions. At the beginning, there was some concern that we were merely describing the upper range of normal manometric pressures. One has to bear in mind, however, that the definition of the nutcracker esophagus was established by identifying patients whose mean peristaltic amplitudes were greater than 2 (or even 3) SD above the mean value of a representative group of controls. This is the appropriate manner to establish normal values and, hence, abnormality. By definition, only 2.5% of the population should be above 2 SD from the mean. Thus, there is the risk that an occasional patient

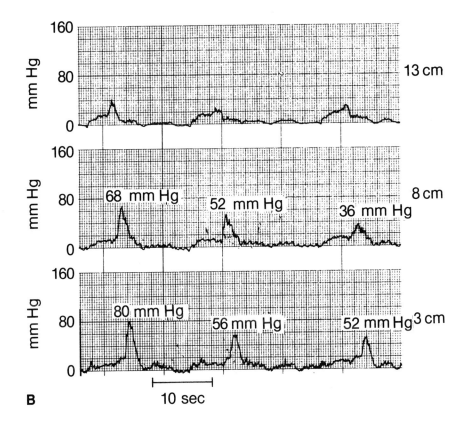

B

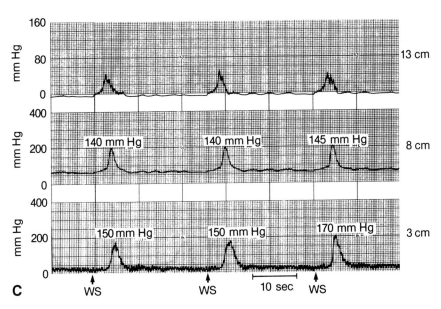

C

TABLE 10.1 Manometric Findings in Patients with Chest Pain[a]

	Seattle[1]	Oklahoma City[3]	Bethesda[4]	New Haven[5]	New Orleans[6]	Winston-Salem[7]
Total patients	?	?	34	112	568	910
Patients with abnormal motility	49	134	22 (65)	48 (43)	114 (20)	255 (28)
Motility diagnosis						
Nutcracker esophagus	20 (41)	37 (28)	10 (45)	13 (27)	54 (38)	122 (48)
Nonspecific esophageal motility disorder	17 (35)	73 (55)	5 (23)		48 (33)	92 (36)
Diffuse esophageal spasm	7 (14)	10 (7)	0	11 (23)	18 (12)	25 (10)
Hypertensive lower esophageal sphincter			5 (23)	11 (23)	17 (12)	11 (4)
Achalasia	5 (10)	14 (10)	2 (9)	13 (27)	7 (5)	5 (2)

[a]Parentheses indicate percentage of patients with abnormality.

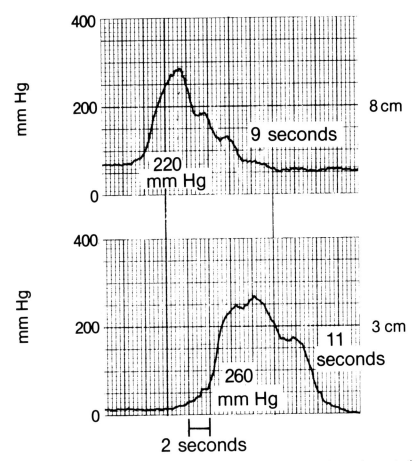

FIGURE 10.2 Motility tracing from another patient with nutcracker esophagus demonstrating the markedly increased duration of peristaltic contractions.

will be called a nutcracker esophagus (1 out of 40) when he is only demonstrating his position in the normal population. It is also important to recognize the differences in contraction amplitudes that can be found in normal individuals in different age groups, as discussed in Chapter 6. This provides the explanation for the change in the pressure level at which we now define the nutcracker esophagus (> 180 mm Hg), as opposed to our initial report of this entity (> 120 mm Hg). When first observed, the pressures in these patients were compared with a group of normal individuals with a mean age in the 20s. Since most of the patients being evaluated for chest pain are in their 40s and 50s, it became clear that normal volunteers in this age range were a more appropriate standard for comparison. This has resulted in our awareness that the nutcracker esophagus should not be diagnosed in patients in these older age groups until mean peristaltic amplitudes exceed 180 mm Hg (see Chapter 6).

Is the Nutcracker Esophagus a True Primary Motility Disorder?

The first evidence comes from the reports of many laboratories, which show that a high percentage of patients being evaluated for chest pain will have this manometric abnormality. In all laboratories that have reported this observation, the percentage was far above the expected 2.5% that might be found in a normal population. This was particularly true in our own series of 910 chest-pain patients, who were studied over a 3-year period.[7] The second piece of evidence also comes from our 3-year study. When looking at the percentage of patients that responded with pain to edrophonium injection (Fig. 10.3), we found that the nutcracker esophagus was the one baseline manometric abnormality that had the highest percentage of positive responses to this drug (see Chapter 11). This evidence supports the concept that the nutcracker esophagus is an important manometric finding that helps to establish the esophagus as a cause of chest pain. Finally, there are now reports appearing in the literature of transition from an initial manometric finding of the nutcracker esophagus to the more traditionally established primary esophageal motility disorder of diffuse esophageal spasm.[8]

Perspectives on the Nutcracker Esophagus

It is important to recognize that there exists some overlap in the classification of patients with primary motility disorders. It is quite likely that many patients with what is now called the nutcracker esophagus were classified as diffuse spasm in the earlier reports. This may be particularly true of those patients who demonstrated excessively prolonged contraction waves. Since the primary hallmark of spasm is the simultaneous nature of the contractions, it is now clear that the large peristaltic waves of the nutcracker esophagus should not be included in this category. Some of this may be perceived as a dialogue between "lumpers" and "splitters," since these patients usually present with similar clinical features (chest pain and/or dysphagia). It has been the decision in our laboratory that every attempt should be made to carefully categorize esophageal motility abnormalities into those groups that seem to separate out as more distinct entities. It is only through establishing more precise descriptions that we can converse in understandable terms and begin to more clearly identify the pathophysiology of these syndromes.

One aspect of the clinical presentation of patients with the nutcracker

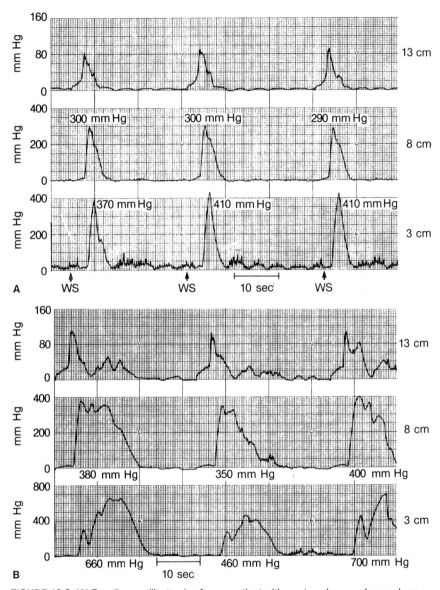

FIGURE 10.3 (A) Baseline motility tracing from a patient with a nutcracker esophagus demonstrating high-amplitude peristaltic contractions. Recording sites located at 13, 8, and 3 cm above the LES. WS, wet swallows. **(B)** Motility tracing from the same patient following the injection of edrophonium (80 μg/kg IV). The marked increase in contraction amplitudes are noted, although the peristaltic nature is maintained. Note change in pressure scale in the distal recording. This patient had reproduction of his typical chest pain during these large contractions.

esophagus is of particular importance. Most of these patients are asymptomatic at the time that their motility abnormality is identified. We have speculated that the manometric findings of the nutcracker esophagus might represent a marker for more severe motility abnormalities occurring at the time of spontaneous pain episodes. Perhaps these patients really do have "spasms" during actual pain events. This same concept might also apply to patients with the hypertensive LES and even the nonspecific esophageal motility disorders (NEMDs) discussed later in this chapter. Thus, it is quite possible that patients who are symptomatic, and who have manometric abnormalities consistent with diffuse esophageal spasm or the other types discussed in this chapter, may truly be part of a spectrum of "spastic disorders of the esophagus" of which classical diffuse spasm would be only one category.

As the concept of the nutcracker esophagus as a clinical entity has evolved, there has been considerable discussion concerning its possible functional importance. It seems unlikely that peristaltic waves of large amplitude should result in any abnormality of esophageal clearance. Since the wave front is peristaltic in these patients, one would anticipate that there would be normal movement of ingested material down the esophagus. Yet there has been evidence of abnormalities of radiolabeled esophageal liquid transit in some of these patients.[9] It is important to note, however, that these studies were not performed at the same time that the patients' motilities were being evaluated. Therefore, it is quite possible that an abnormal peristaltic pattern actually occurred at the time of the radionuclide study. In our laboratory, we have performed simultaneous studies of radionuclide esophageal transit and esophageal manometry in normal subjects and in patients with the nutcracker esophagus. These studies revealed that esophageal liquid transit is normal whenever the contraction wave has a peristaltic wavefront, irrespective of the amplitude or duration of the contractile wave or the presence of repetitive peaks.[10]

THE HYPERTENSIVE LOWER ESOPHAGEAL SPHINCTER

The presence of an excessively high resting LES pressure in patients with esophageal symptoms was first described in 1960 by Code et al at the Mayo Clinic.[11] Although many of the patients had other evidence of esophageal motility abnormalities (particularly diffuse spasm), approximately 50% of these patients showed only isolated abnormalities of the LES. These patients were characterized by increased resting LES pressures associated with normal LES relaxation and normal peristalsis. A subsequent report of a similar finding was made by Garrett and Godwin.[12] In this report, the patients also had excessively large and prolonged contractions of the sphincter following relaxation, a phenomenon called the "hypercontracting or hyperreacting sphincter." It is quite likely that many of these patients, particularly those with the "hypercontracting" sphincter, belong to the subsequently described motility disorder, the nutcracker esophagus.

It is interesting that in both of these early reports approximately 3 out of 4 of the patients had chest pain, often similar to that occurring with cardiac disease. Dysphagia was also present in some patients. It is not clear why this single manometric finding might produce these symptoms. The comments made above about the functional importance of the nutcracker esophagus might also apply to patients with the hypertensive LES. It seems unlikely that a high resting LES pressure, which relaxes normally on swallowing and is associated with a normal peristaltic wave, should result in a functional impairment of esophageal transit. Like the nutcracker esophagus, it is quite likely that this finding may only represent an important manometric marker for the presence of intermittent motility abnormalities of greater severity at the time that the patients are symptomatic. A patient with a hypertensive LES, whose dysphagia was so severe that pneumatic dilatation was performed to relieve the symptom, was recently described.[13]

In the studies that are currently being performed in patients with noncardiac chest pain, a small percentage of patients demonstrate the phenomenon of the hypertensive LES. In our laboratory, this is defined by LES pressure exceeding 2 SD above the normal range. This is specifically identified by pressures greater than 45 mm Hg. Figure 10.4 is a motility tracing from a patient who has been seen over a period of three years for recurring noncardiac chest pain. On two occasions, separated by two years, the patient demonstrated the isolated finding of the hypertensive LES, in the range of 60 to 70 mm Hg.

NONSPECIFIC ESOPHAGEAL MOTILITY DISORDERS

When evaluating large numbers of patients for potential esophageal motility abnormalities, one frequently finds the presence of esophageal contraction patterns that are outside of the range of normal findings, yet do not readily fit into the more clearly defined categories of the other primary motility disorders. This is particularly true when studying groups of patients with unexplained chest pain. It is obviously essential that a clear understanding of the spectrum of normal esophageal motility findings be available before one can even begin to categorize patients as NEMDs (see Chapter 6). Table 10.2

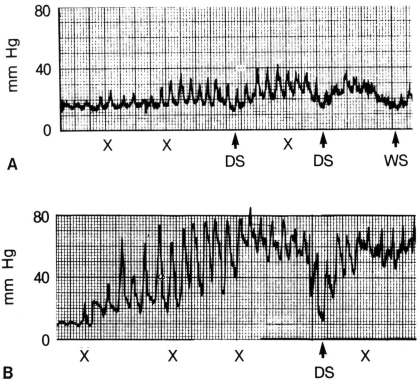

FIGURE 10.4 Lower esophageal sphincter pressure recording during station pull-through (SPT) from a normal subject **(A)** and a patient with the hypertensive LES **(B)**. DS, dry swallow; WS, wet swallow; X, tube moved up 0.5 cm.

summarizes the types of motility findings seen in our laboratory that are considered to be abnormal and result in the classification of an NEMD. These patterns run a broad spectrum of abnormalities and the true clinical significance of these findings remains to be discovered. In some cases, the finding of an NEMD is clearly a precursor to the eventual development of a more defined primary motility disorder. We have seen at least one patient over the years who has shown a transition from NEMD to diffuse esophageal spasm to classic achalasia.

It should be noted that a similar attempt at classification has been published by Clouse and Staiano.[14] Although some of the terms are different, the classification proposed by them is quite similar to that used in our laboratory. Thus, their finding of high-amplitude and/or long-duration contraction abnormalities would be consistent with the nutcracker esophagus.

TABLE 10.2 Manometric Criteria for Primary Esophageal Motility Disorders

Achalasia (see Chapter 8)
Diffuse esophageal spasm (see Chapter 9)
Nutcracker esophagus
    Peristaltic waves of high amplitude ($\bar{x}$: > 180 mm Hg)
    May also be prolonged duration ($\bar{x}$: > 6.0 sec)
    Normal peristaltic progression
Hypertensive lower esophageal sphincter (LES)
    Resting LES pressure > 45 mm Hg
    Normal LES relaxation
    Normal peristaltic progression
Nonspecific esophageal motility disorder (any combination of the following)
    Increased nontransmitted contractions ($\geqq$ 20% of wet swallows)
    Triple-peaked contractions
    Retrograde contractions
    Low-amplitude contractions (< 30 mm Hg)
    Isolated, incomplete LES relaxation
    Prolonged-duration peristaltic waves (> 6 sec)

The abnormal waveforms and triple-peaked waves in this classification would be NEMDs or diffuse esophageal spasm, depending on whether or not there were simultaneous contraction abnormalities.

REFERENCES

1. Brand DL, Martin D, Pope CE: Esophageal manometrics in patients with anginal type chest pain. *Am J Dig Dis* 1977;23:300–304.
2. Benjamin SB, Gerhardt DC, Castell DO: High amplitude peristaltic contractions associated with chest pain and/or dysphagia. *Gastroenterology* 1979;77:478–483.
3. Orr WC, Robinson MG: Hypertensive peristalsis in the pathogenesis of chest pain. *Am J Gastroenterol* 1982;77:604–607.
4. Benjamin SB, Richter JE, Cordova CM, et al: Prospective manometric evaluation with pharmacologic provocation of patients with suspected esophageal motility dysfunction. *Gastroenterology* 1983;84:893–901.
5. Traube M, Abibi R, McCallum RW: High amplitude peristaltic esophageal contractions associated with chest pain. *JAMA* 1983;250:2655–2659.
6. Herrington JP, Burns TW, Balart LA: Chest pain and dysphagia in patients with prolonged peristaltic contractile duration of the esophagus. *Dig Dis Sci* 1984;29:134–140.
7. Katz PO, Dalton CB, Wu WC, et al: Esophageal testing of patients with non-cardiac chest pain or dysphagia. *Ann Intern Med* 1987;106:593–597.
8. Narducci F, Bassotti G, Gaburri M, et al: Transition from nutcracker esophagus to diffuse esophageal spasm. *Am J Gastroenterol* 1985;80:242–244.
9. Benjamin SB, O'Donnell JR, Hancock J, et al: Prolonged radionuclide transit in "nutcracker esophagus." *Dig Dis Sci* 1983;28:775–779.

10. Richter JE, Blackwell JN, Wu WC, et al: Relationship of radionuclide liquid bolus transport and esophageal manometry. *J Lab Clin Med* 1987;109:217–224.
11. Code CF, Schlegel JF, Kelley ML, et al: Hypertensive gastroesophageal sphincter. *Proc Mayo Clinic* 1960;35:391–399.
12. Garrett JM, Godwin DH: Gastroesophageal hypercontracting sphincter. *JAMA* 1969;208:992–998.
13. Traube M, Lagarde S, McCallum RW: Isolated hypertensive lower esophageal sphincter: treatment of a resistant case by pneumatic dilatation. *J Clin Gastroenterol* 1984;6:139–142.
14. Clouse RE, Staiano A: Contraction abnormalities of the esophageal body in patients referred for manometry. *Dig Dis Sci* 1983;28:784–791.

CHAPTER 11

Noncardiac Chest Pain
Use of Esophageal
Manometry and Provocative Tests

Joel E. Richter, MD, FACP

Noncardiac chest pain is a vexing diagnostic problem. The common innervation of the heart and esophagus permits esophageal disorders to mimic the chest pain produced by coronary artery disease. The magnitude of this medical problem is striking. Approximately 500,000 coronary angiograms are performed in the United States each year.[1] Of these, it is estimated that 10% to 30% are normal, resulting in as many as 150,000 new patients having unexplained—and therefore possibly esophageal—chest pain diagnosed each year.[2] Recent reports estimate that up to 60% of patients with noncardiac chest pain may have an identifiable esophageal abnormality.[3-7] Accepting a 50% estimate as correct, one can anticipate 75,000 new cases of esophageal chest pain per year.

The major potential mechanisms for esophageal pain are stimulation of pain receptors in the esophageal mucosa and changes in esophageal wall tension, which stimulates mechanoreceptors. Although abnormalities in esophageal motility may be evoked by acid perfusion,[8] dysmotility is not usually found during pain production.[9] Thus, the demonstration of pain during intraesophageal acid perfusion is most likely related to stimulation of acid-sensitive chemoreceptors in the esophageal mucosa. Chest pain secondary to excessive esophageal contractions or esophageal spasms might be reasonably explained on the basis of changes in esophageal wall tension stimulating mechanoreceptors. A potential method of testing this hypothesis would involve pharmacologic stimulation of increased esophageal contractile activity in an attempt to reproduce symptoms in pain-prone patients. The issue is further confounded by the possibility that patients with noncardiac chest pain may have lower pain thresholds[10] as a result of emotional disorders or stress.[11,12] Thus, these patients may only perceive pain abnormally in response to physiologic events.

INITIAL EVALUATION: RULE OUT HEART DISEASE

The prevalence of cardiac and esophageal diseases increases as the population grows older.[13] Therefore, both problems may co-exist in chest-pain patients and complicate diagnostic evaluations. The clinical history and physical examination are frequently not helpful. Features that may suggest esophageal rather than cardiac pain include: an atypical response to exercise; pain that continues for hours; retrosternal pain without lateral radiation; pain that interrupts sleep or is meal related; pain relieved with antacids; or the presence of associated esophageal symptoms, including heartburn, dysphagia, or regurgitation. However, as many as 50% of patients with cardiac pain may have these characteristics of esophageal pain; therefore, clinical features do not permit reliable discrimination between the two groups.[14] In younger patients (< 40 years) without a family history of heart disease, cardiac problems can usually be excluded by a normal exercise stress test and echocardiogram. Older patients will generally need coronary angiography with possible ergonovine testing to exclude significant cardiac disease. After such a negative evaluation, these patients can be reassured that their heart is normal and that their noncardiac chest pains will not lead to increased cardiac events or death.[15] Despite these reassurances, a significant number continue to experience chest pain, continue to think they have heart disease, have limited lifestyles, and remain unable to work.[16]

After cardiac disease has been ruled out, the next step in our evaluation is barium studies or endoscopy to evaluate the upper gastrointestinal (GI) tract. These studies may reveal an unusual cause of chest pain, such as an esophageal or gastric cancer or peptic ulcerations presenting with atypical pain patterns. More commonly, reflux esophagitis is found, which suggests a *probable* esophageal cause for the chest pain. A gallbladder study may also be useful, because biliary pain sometimes results in pain referred to the lower chest. A point to remember is that this study may show otherwise "silent" gallstones, and the mere finding of gallstones does not prove the cause of pain.

ESOPHAGEAL TESTING

Esophageal testing for noncardiac chest pain is the primary indication for referrals to our esophageal laboratory. Over the last 3 years, we have evaluated 1250 patients with esophageal manometry for the following primary complaints: noncardiac chest pain (72%), dysphagia (20%), and miscellaneous (ie, prior to anti-reflux surgery or exclude collagen vascular diseases; 8%). Esophageal testing should include esophageal manometry and various provocative tests, particularly in patients with noncardiac chest pain.

ESOPHAGEAL MANOMETRY

Esophageal motility disorders have been associated with noncardiac chest pain, but may be less frequent than commonly thought. There is broad disparity among previously reported series,[3,7,17] with the prevalence ranging from 6% to 68%. We recently reviewed our 3-year experience with 910 patients referred for evaluation of noncardiac chest pain.[18] Only 255 of these patients (28%) had esophageal motility disorders, compared to the 132 out of 251 patients (53%) referred for evaluation of dysphagia (Fig. 11.1). In agreement with other recent series,[3,17,19,20] the nutcracker esophagus (48%) was

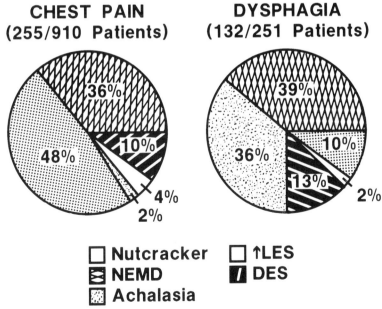

FIGURE 11.1 Pie diagram comparing incidence of esophageal motility disorders in patients with noncardiac chest pain (left) and dysphagia (right). NEMD, nonspecific esophageal motility disorder; ↑LES, hypertensive lower esophageal sphincter; DES, diffuse esophageal spasm.

clearly the most common motility disorder found in patients with noncardiac chest pain, while classic diffuse esophageal spasm (10%) was an infrequent finding. Nonspecific esophageal motility disorders (NEMDs; 36%), hypertensive lower esophageal sphincter ($\uparrow$ LES, 4%), and achalasia (2%) completed the other identifiable motility disorders. In contrast, achalasia (39%) was the most common motility diagnosis in patients with dysphagia, while nutcracker esophagus (10%) was an infrequent finding (Fig. 11.1). All manometric diagnoses, particularly nutcracker esophagus and NEMD, were defined in our laboratory as being at least 2 SD away from mean values in a group of 95 normal adults.

The documentation of the presence of an esophageal motility disorder *does not* conclusively prove that it is the source of the patient's chest pain. In fact, esophageal motility studies of many patients with noncardiac chest pain show baseline abnormalities at a time when they are pain-free. The spontaneous onset of chest pain with abnormal esophageal motility is a rare occurrence in our laboratory. Therefore, we believe the presence of an esophageal motility disorder only suggests the esophagus is a *probable* source of chest pain. Further provocative testing is required to identify the esophagus as a *definite* cause of chest pain.

PROVOCATIVE TESTS
Historical Perspectives

A major goal of investigators has been to find methods for correlating esophageal dysfunction with chest pain. Unlike the coronary angiogram in ischemic heart disease, studies in noncardiac chest pain have been hampered by the lack of a "gold standard" for diagnosing esophageal chest pain. Nevertheless, a useful approach is to provoke the functional esophageal abnormalities that might result in pain — an esophageal "stress test." Provocative agents have included ice-water swallows[21,22]; intraesophageal acid perfusion[23]; and systemic injections of bethanechol,[24] edrophonium,[25,26] ergonovine,[25,27] and pentagastrin.[28] Studies with ice-water swallows have been limited to case reports, but do suggest that cold-induced pain is not secondary to esophageal spasm.[29] The α-adrenergic stimulant ergonovine has been the drug most extensively studied and may replicate esophageal chest pain in 22%–60% of patients.[27,30,31,32] Ergonovine, however, is a nonspecific stimulant (it does induce coronary spasm), may cause chest pain in healthy controls, and is associated with a high incidence of side effects, particularly cardiac arrythmias.[27,32] Furthermore, the only available comparison study found ergonovine no better than edrophonium in provoking chest pain and abnormal contractile activity in a group of patients with high-amplitude esophageal contractions.[25] Pentagastrin (6 μg/kg SC) and bethanechol (40 μg/kg SC) have minimal cardiac toxicity, but in a recent comparison study replicated esophageal chest pain in only 6% and 12% of patients, respectively.[17] Other reports, however, suggest that higher doses (50 μg/kg SC) and repeated injections of bethanechol may reproduce esophageal chest pain in 33% to 77% of symptomatic patients.[33,34] At these higher doses, the uncomfortable side effects and pain from subcutaneous injections of bethanechol may limit its clinical usefulness. As discussed in the following two sections, we have found intraesophageal acid perfusion and edrophonium (Tensilon) to be the best and safest provocative tests for routine use in the clinical esophageal laboratory.

Acid-Perfusion (Bernstein) Test

Since its introduction in 1958 by Bernstein and Baker,[23] esophageal acid perfusion has been widely accepted and used as a clinical test for gastroesophageal (GE) reflux disease. It is a simple test that has both a sensitivity and a specificity of approximately 80%.[35] It also may be a useful provocative test in patients with GE reflux disease, who present primarily with chest pains rather than heartburn. In our experience with 910 noncardiac chest-pain patients, 61 (7%) patients had the acid-perfusion test reproduce their chest pains.

The acid-perfusion test is a simple procedure that we usually perform with the patient in the supine position after the manometry study and before the edrophonium provocation test. There are several published methods of procedures, but the ideal method is to alternate saline with dilute acid (0.1 N HCl) to obtain a placebolike control. Both solutions are infused into the distal esophagus at the rate of 6 to 8 mL/min. The saline should not cause the chest pain; the acid should replicate the patient's identical complaints of chest pain to be called a positive test. It is preferable to alternately infuse acid and saline at least twice to try to make the chest pain come and go.

Edrophonium (Tensilon) Test

Edrophonium hydrochloride, a cholinesterase inhibitor used in the diagnosis of myasthenia gravis, is a relatively safe and specific provocative test for esophageal chest pain. At a dose of 80 μg/kg IV, it produces a pharmacologic increase in the amplitude and duration of esophageal contractions, both in normals and in patients with disorders of esophageal motility (Fig. 11.2). In several series,[17,26] edrophonium has provoked chest pain in 18%–30% of noncardiac chest-pain patients but *not* in over 150 asymptomatic volunteers. It was initially hoped that the manometric response to edrophonium

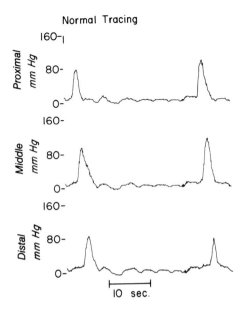

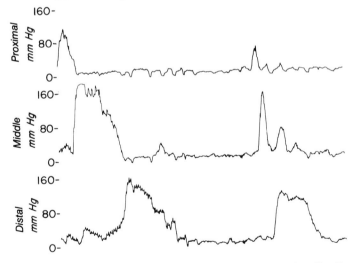

FIGURE 11.2 Manometry tracing at top demonstrates normal esophageal motility. Tracing at bottom demonstrates typical edrophonium response, showing markedly increased amplitude and duration of esophageal contractions. Note that peristalsis persists after the administration of edrophonium.

might characterize patients with esophageal chest pain and give some clues to the pathogenesis of their pain. Unfortunately, healthy control subjects and patients with noncardiac chest pain, regardless of their edrophonium pain response, develop as a group, the same manometric response to edrophonium (Fig. 11.3).[26] Therefore, as in the acid-perfusion test, the key endpoint for a positive edrophonium test is *pain*, rather than a specific change in esophageal motility. Aside from occasional lightheadedness, nausea, or abdominal cramps, we have seen no important side effects after edrophonium and no patients have required treatment with atropine for reversal of side effects. Unlike ergonovine, edrophonium does not potentially promote myocardial ischemia by increasing heart rate or systolic blood pressure, nor does it reduce coronary blood flow by constricting epicardial vessels.[26]

In our laboratory, a placebo-controlled edrophonium provocation test is done for all patients with noncardiac chest pain after baseline manometry and the acid-perfusion test. A placebo (1 mL of 0.9% normal saline) and edrophonium (80 μg/kg) are consecutively administered intravenously by rapid bolus infusion, in an order unknown to the patient. Immediately after each injection, ten 5-mL water swallows are given over 5 min and the patient is asked about chest pain and the similarities of symptoms to those of their chronic pain syndrome. A positive test is defined as replication of the patient's chest pain within 5 min, only after the edrophonium injection. An atypical test result (pain after placebo or both placebo and edrophonium) may occur ($\sim$ 5%), but is considered nondiagnostic for esophageal chest pain. Since the esophageal motility response does not characterize edrophonium-positive patients, the test can also be performed in the office without esophageal manometry.

Our Clinical Experience with Manometry and Provocative Tests in the Evaluation of Noncardiac Chest Pain

In our recent review of 910 patients with noncardiac chest pain,[18] 61 (7%) patients had positive acid-perfusion tests and 210 (23%) positive edrophonium tests. When patients having positives for both provocative tests are counted as a single positive, 243 out of 910 (27%) patients had their chest pain reproduced in the laboratory and were considered to have a *definite* esophageal source for their pain (Fig. 11.4). Patients with baseline motility disorders were as likely to have chest pain with provocative testing (25%) as patients with normal motility (27%). Patients with nutcracker esophagus had a higher frequency of positive provocative tests compared to normals (34% versus 27%, $P = 0.07$) and patients with other motility disorders (34% versus 16%, $P < 0.05$). The combination of patients with *definite* esophageal chest pain (27%) and *probable* esophageal pain [abnormal manometry only; 192

150

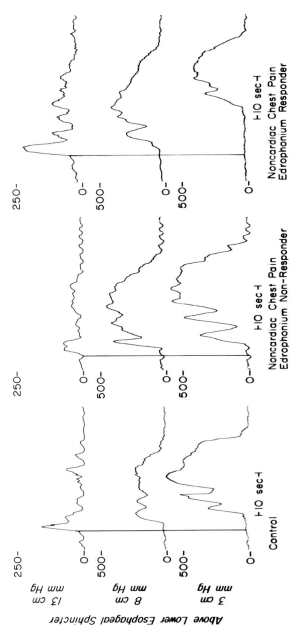

FIGURE 11.3 Individual esophageal contractile activity after IV injection of edrophonium (80 μg/kg body weight) does not distinguish control subjects, patients with noncardiac chest pain who do not develop pain after edrophonium administration, and patients with noncardiac chest pain in whom edrophonium replicates their pain.

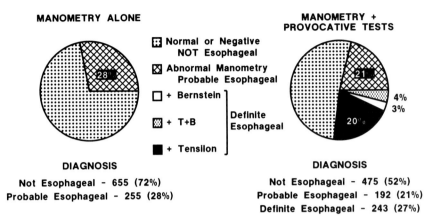

MANOMETRY ALONE

MANOMETRY +
PROVOCATIVE TESTS

▦ Normal or Negative
  NOT Esophageal

▨ Abnormal Manometry
  Probable Esophageal

☐ + Bernstein ⎫
              ⎪ Definite
▨ + T+B   ⎬ Esophageal
              ⎪
■ + Tensilon ⎭

4%
3%

DIAGNOSIS

Not Esophageal - 655 (72%)
Probable Esophageal - 255 (28%)

DIAGNOSIS

Not Esophageal - 475 (52%)
Probable Esophageal - 192 (21%)
Definite Esophageal - 243 (27%)

FIGURE 11.4 Pie diagram illustrating diagnostic yield of esophageal testing in 910 patients with noncardiac chest pain. Esophageal manometry alone is compared with manometry and provocative tests. T + B, Tensilon and Bernstein tests.

out of 910 (21%) patients] gives an overall diagnostic yield of 48% for our esophageal laboratory (Fig. 11.4). Therefore, provocative testing compliments esophageal manometry alone and nearly doubles our diagnostic yield of esophageal chest pain. These patients can now be given an alternative cause for their chest pain and follow-up studies suggest they are less likely to be disabled by their pain or to require continued use of health care resources.[36]

FUTURE DEVELOPMENTS
Graded Esophageal Balloon Distention

Balloon distention of the esophagus was one of the earliest methods attempted to distinguish esophageal and cardiac chest pain.[37] Subsequently, the electrocardiogram (ECG) was found to be a more sensitive test for cardiac chest pain. We have recently "rediscovered" balloon distention as a possible provocation test for esophageal chest pain.[10,38] A polyvinyl balloon (length: 30 mm; maximum diameter after 10-cc distention: 25mm) was positioned 10 cm above the LES and inflated with 1-cc increments of air to a total volume of 10 cc. Pain occurred in 28 out of 50 (56%) noncardiac chest-pain patients and 6 out of 30 (20%) healthy volunteers ($P < 0.005$). Symptoms were unassociated with ECG changes and resolved immediately upon balloon decompression. Chest-pain patients were observed to have lowered pain threshold for esophageal distention, since 24 out of 28 patients had chest pain at ≤ 8-cc distention, while all volunteers with pain noted it at

≥ 9-cc distention. For this reason, 8 cc was considered our diagnostic cutoff. Graded esophageal balloon distention was subsequently compared to acid perfusion and edrophonium tests (Fig. 11.5). These conventional tests reproduced pain in only 12 (24%) patients. Positive balloon studies occurred in 11 of these patients and identified an additional 13 patients, thus increasing the diagnostic yield from 24% to 48%. Only one of 26 (4%) balloon-negative patients had a positive acid-perfusion or edrophonium test. This new provocative test offers great promise. A commercially produced balloon and automated infusion system (Wilson-Cook Medical Inc., Winston-Salem, NC) should be available in late 1987.

Ambulatory 24-Hour pH and Pressure Monitoring

Ambulatory pH monitors are currently available and have been very useful in the evaluation of difficult cases of suspected GE reflux disease. The devel-

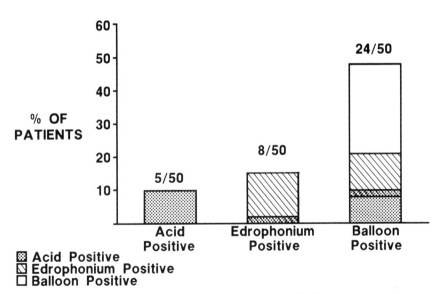

FIGURE 11.5 Comparison of chest-pain response with graded balloon distention to conventional esophageal provocative tests. Acid-perfusion produced pain in 5 out of 50 (10%) patients. Edrophonium produced pain in 8 out of 50 (16%) patients. One patient had positives for both the acid and edrophonium tests. Overall, the combination of conventional tests identified the esophagus as a definite cause of chest pain in 12 out of 50 (24%) patients. A positive balloon study occurred in 11 of these patients as well as in an additional 13. Therefore, the diagnostic yield of balloon distention alone was 48% (24 out of 50 patients).

opment of a system to simultaneously measure both esophageal pH and motility would permit monitoring of several episodes of spontaneously occurring chest pain throughout the day. We have recently tested a prototype system and studied it in 22 noncardiac chest-pain patients with 92 spontaneous episodes of chest pain.[39] Overall, 13 out of 22 patients (59%) had at least one chest-pain event associated with normal esophageal pH or motility. Thirty-three chest pain episodes (36%) were correlated with abnormal motility (11 events), pH ≤ 4 (18 events), or both (4 events), but 59 chest-pain events (64%) were not associated with abnormal esophageal activity. Patients could not distinguish chest-pain episodes arising from abnormal motility or pH from episodes not associated with abnormal esophageal activity. Using a comparable pressure and pH system, a Belgian group has recently reported a similar series of patients but identified an esophageal cause of chest pain in only 35% of their patients.[40]

REFERENCES

1. Kennedy RH, Kennedy MA, Frye RL, et al: Cardiac catherization and cardiac surgical facilities. *N Engl J Med* 1982;307:986–993.
2. Kemp HG, Vokonas PS, Cohn PF, et al: The anginal syndrome associated with normal coronary arteriograms. *Am J Med* 1973;54:735–742.
3. Brand DL, Martin D, Pope CE: Esophageal manometries in patients with angina-like chest pain. *Dig Dis Sci* 1977;4:300–304.
4. Kline M, Chessne R, Studevant RAL, et al: Esophageal disease in patients with angina-like chest pain. *Am J Gastroenterol* 1981;75:116–123.
5. Fergunson SC, Hodges K, Hersh T, et al: Esophageal manometry in patients with chest pain and normal coronary arteriograms. *Am J Gastroenterol* 1981;75:124–127.
6. DeMeester TR, O'Sullivan GC, Bermudez G, et al: Esophageal function in patients with angina-type chest pain and normal coronary angiograms. *Ann Surg* 1982;196:488–498.
7. Alban-Davies H, Jones DB, Rhoades J: Esophageal angina as the cause of chest pain. *JAMA* 1982;248:2274–2278.
8. Siegal CI, Hendrix TR: Esophageal motor abnormalities induced by acid perfusion in patients with heartburn. *J Clin Invest* 1963;42:689–695.
9. Richter JE, Johns DN, Wu WC, et al: Are esophageal motility abnormalities produced during the intraesophageal acid perfusion test? *JAMA* 1985;253:1914–1917.
10. Richter JE, Barish CF, Castell DO: Abnormal sensory perception in patients with esophageal chest pain. *Gastroenterology* 1986;91:845–852.
11. Clouse RE, Lustman PJ: Psychiatric illness and contraction abnormalities of the esophagus. *N Engl J Med* 1983;309:1337–1342.
12. Richter JE, Obrecht WF, Bradley LA, et al: Psychological comparison of patients with nutcracker esophagus and irritable bowel syndrome. *Dig Dis Sci* 1986;31:131–138.
13. Svensson O, Stenport G, Tibbling L, et al: Oesophageal function and coronary angiogram in patients with disabling chest pain. *Acta Med Scand* 1978;204:173–178.

14. Alban-Davies H, Jones DB, Rhodes J, et al: Angina-like esophageal pain: differentiation from cardiac pain by history. *J Clin Gastroenterol* 1985;7:477–481.
15. Wielgasz AT, Fletcher RH, McCants CB, et al: Unimproved chest pain in patients with minimal or no coronary disease: A behavioral phenomenon. *Am Heart J* 1984;108:67–72.
16. Ockene IS, Shay MJ, Alpert JS, et al: Unexplained chest pain in patients with normal coronary arteriograms. A follow-up study of functional status. *New Engl J Med* 1980;303:1249–1252.
17. Benjamin SB, Richter JE, Cordova CM, et al: Prospective manometric evaluation with pharmacologic provocation of patients with suspected esophageal motility dysfunction. *Gastroenterology* 1983;84:893–901.
18. Katz PO, Dalton CB, Richter JE, et al: Esophageal testing of patients with non-cardiac chest pain and/or dysphagia. Results of a three year experience with 1161 patients. *Ann Intern Med* 1987;106:593–597.
19. Clouse RE, Staiano A: Contraction abnormalities of the esophageal body in patients referred for manometry; a new approach to manometric classification. *Dig Dis Sci* 1983;28:784–791.
20. Traube M, Albibi R, McCallum RW: High amplitude esophageal contractions associated with chest pain. *JAMA* 1983;250:2655–2659.
21. Respess JC, Inglefinger FJ, Kramer P: Effect of cold on esophageal motor function. *Am J Med* 1952;20:955.
22. Catalano CJ, Bozymski EM, Orlando RC: Temperature-dependent symptoms in a patient with esophageal motor disease. *Gastroenterology* 1983;85:1407–1410.
23. Bernstein LM, Baker LA: A clinical test for esophagitis. *Gastroenterology* 1958;34:760–781.
24. Mellow M. Symptomatic diffuse esophageal spasm: manometric follow-up and response to cholinergic stimulation and cholinesterase inhibition. *Gastroenterology* 1977;73:237–240.
25. London RL, Ouyang A, Snape WJ, et al: Provocation of esophageal pain by ergonovine or edrophonium. *Gastroenterology* 1981;81:10–14.
26. Richter JE, Hackshaw BT, Wu WC: Edrophonium: a useful provocative test for esophageal chest pain. *Ann Intern Med* 1985;103:14–21.
27. Alban-Davies H, Kaye MD, Rhodes J, et al: Diagnosis of esophageal spasm by ergometrine provocation. *Gut* 1982;23:89–97.
28. Orlando RC, Bozymski EM: The effect of pentagastrin in achalasia and diffuse esophageal spasm. *Gastroenterology* 1979;77:472–477.
29. Meyer GW, Castell DO: Human esophageal response during chest pain induced by swallowing cold liquids. *JAMA* 1981;246:2057–2059.
30. Eastwood GL, Weiner BH, Dickerson WJ: Use of ergonovine to identify esophageal spasm in patients with chest pain. *Ann Intern Med* 1981;94:768–771.
31. Koch KL, Curry RC, Feldman RL, et al: Ergonovine-induced esophageal spasm in patients with chest pain resembling angina pectoris. *Dig Dis Sci* 1982;27:1073–1080.
32. Myers D: Ergonovine provocation of coronary artery spasm. *Cardiovasc Rev Resp* 1982;3:855–863.
33. Nostrant TT, Sams JS, Huber T: Bethanechol increases the diagnostic yield in patients with esophageal chest pain. *Gastroenterology* 1986;91:1141–1146.
34. Cole MJ, Paterson WA, Beck IT, et al: The effect of acid and bethanechol stimulation in patients with symptomatic hypertensive peristaltic (nutcracker) esophagus. *J Clin Gastroenterol* 1986;8:223–229.
35. Richter JE, Castell DO: Gastroesophageal reflux. Pathogenesis, diagnosis and therapy. *Ann Intern Med* 1982;97:93–103.
36. Ward BW, Wu WC, Richter JE, et al: Long-term follow-up of symptomatic status of patients with noncardiac chest pain: Is diagnosis of esophageal etiology helpful? *Am J Gastroenterol* 1987;82:215–218.

37. Kramer P, Hollander W: Comparison of experimental esophageal pain with clinical pain of angina pectoris and esophageal disease. *Gastroenterology* 1955;29:719–743.
38. Barish CF, Castell DO, Richter JE: Graded esophageal balloon distention: a new provocation test for non-cardiac chest pain. *Dig Dis Sci* 1986;31:1292–1298.
39. Peters LJ, Maas LC, Dalton CB, et al: Twenty-four hour ambulatory combined esophageal motility/pH monitoring in evaluation of non-cardiac chest pain (abstr). *Gastroenterology* 1986;90:1584A.
40. Janssens J, Vantrappen G, Ghillebert G: Twenty-four hour recording of esophageal pressure and pH in patients with noncardiac chest pain. *Gastroenterology* 1986;90:1978–1984.

Exogenous Factors
Affecting Esophageal Motility

Thomas P. McMahon, MD

A variety of substances used in everyday life, including various foods, alcohol, tobacco-containing products, and drugs, have been investigated for their effects on the esophagus. This chapter will review the reported effects of these substances on esophageal manometric parameters.

TOBACCO-CONTAINING PRODUCTS

Cigarette smoking has been shown to produce a number of deleterious effects on the esophagus, which may predispose to the development of gastroesophageal reflux disease (GERD). A variety of mechanisms by which cigarette smoking may contribute to GERD have been proposed and are summarized in Table 12.1.

Manometric studies during cigarette smoking have demonstrated a significant decrease in lower esophageal sphincter (LES) pressure, ranging from 19%–42%.[1-3] Figure 12.1 illustrates LES pressure changes in six volunteers before and during smoking. In contrast, puffing on an unlit cigarette did not

TABLE 12.1 Motility Abnormalities and Other Effects of Smoking that May Contribute to Gastroesophageal Reflux Disease

Decreased lower esophageal sphincter pressure
Impaired esophageal clearance
Decreased mucosal resistance
More injurious refluxate
Diminished acid-suppressing effect of H_2 blockers

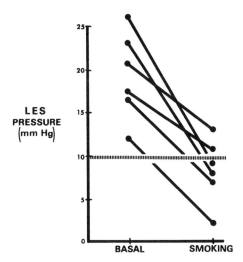

FIGURE 12.1 Lower esophageal sphincter (LES) pressure for six volunteer subjects basally and during cigarette smoking. The hatched line indicates separation between an effective (> 10 mm Hg) and an incompetent (< 10 mm Hg) LES.

alter LES pressure in any of these studies. Nicotine infused intravenously in the opossum will also result in a marked decrease in LES pressure.[4] In addition, a fall in sphincter pressure can also occur after smokeless nicotine ingestion (Nicorette gum).

We have evaluated the effects of a variety of nicotine-containing products on esophageal peristalsis.[5] Compared to chewing gum (placebo) neither cigarette smoking, Nicorette gum, nor Skoal Bandit had any effect on the amplitude, duration, or velocity of the peristaltic wave. None of the test substances produced a motility abnormality. There is, however, some evidence that smoking will impair esophageal clearance.[6]

ALCOHOL

The acute administration of intoxicating amounts of ethanol by the oral or intravenous route has been found to produce transient impairment of esophageal motor function in normal human volunteers.[7] Abnormalities in the esophageal body included decreased incidence of primary peristalsis and frequent simultaneous nonpropulsive contractions following wet swallows. There were no changes in the velocity, amplitude, or duration of the peristaltic wave. LES pressure was reduced after both oral and intravenous ethanol.

In chronic alcoholics with peripheral neuropathy, a diminution of primary peristalsis, with a corresponding increase in nonperistaltic contractions, has been reported.[8]

FOOD

A variety of foods have been evaluated for their effects on the esophagus. Most studies have evaluated the effects of these foods on LES pressure. A summary of these studies is outlined in Table 12.2.

Chocolate has been shown to lower LES pressure. This effect might be attributed to the high fat content of most chocolate preparations. However, defatted chocolate syrup also lowers LES pressure in a dose-dependent fashion (Fig. 12.2). This effect is most likely caused by the high chocolate content of methyl xanthine (theobromine), which inhibits phosphodiesterase, resulting in increased intracellular cyclic AMP (cAMP). Increased levels of cAMP have a relaxant effect on the smooth muscle of the gastrointestinal tract.[9]

Volunteer studies with equal-calorie test meals have shown significant decreases of LES pressure after fat ingestion and augmentation of sphincter pressures after protein. Glucose produced no pressure change.[10] Carminatives, including peppermint and spearmint, have been shown to result in decreased LES pressure.[11]

The effects of coffee on the esophagus are less clear. Initial studies with caffeine alone suggested minimal decrease in LES pressure.[12] A subsequent study found that brewed regular and decaffeinated coffee both increased LES pressure and augmented acid production, while caffeine alone had no effect on sphincter pressure.[13] Yet another study reached opposite conclusions, finding that one cup of instant caffeinated coffee decreased LES pressure over 60 min in healthy volunteers.[14] It has been subsequently shown that

TABLE 12.2 Effects of Foods on Esophageal Function

Decrease LES pressure
  Fat
  Chocolate
  Peppermint
  Alcohol
Increase LES pressure
  Protein
  Coffee (?)
Diminish or disorder peristalsis
  Alcohol
  Ice cream
Cause direct mucosal irritation
  Orange juice
  Spicy tomato juice
  Coffee

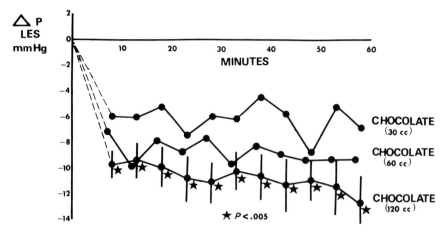

FIGURE 12.2 Effects of different doses of ingested chocolate syrup on lower esophageal sphincter (LES) pressures in human volunteers. Each dot represents mean change in pressure (ΔP) from basal value for 10 subjects. Vertical lines, ± 1 SE, and stars indicate significant changes from baseline mean pressure ($P < 0.005$).

caffeinated coffee has no significant effect on LES pressure in the fasting or postprandial state.[15] Interpreting these conflicting data is difficult.

Another mechanism by which coffee may potentiate reflux symptoms without altering LES pressure in patients with esophageal-acid sensitivity secondary to inflamed esophageal mucosa has been proposed. Citrus juices and tomato products (bases in many spicy products) may exert a similar effect (Table 12.2). While generally not affecting LES pressure, these food substances have a direct pH-independent irritating effect on inflamed esophageal mucosa.[16] This effect may be related to the high osmolality of these products.[17]

TEMPERATURE

The effect of the ingestion of cold liquids on the esophagus was initially reported by Winship et al.[18] Normal volunteers given ice water were found to develop sharply diminished frequency of peristalsis in the proximal and distal esophagus, decreased wave velocity, and decreased wave duration in the distal esophagus. Meyer and Castell later studied the response to swallowing soft ice cream in normal volunteers.[19] Decreased peristaltic amplitudes occurred in the mid- and distal esophagus. When ice cream was ingested rapidly until chest pain was produced, complete absence of contractions in the distal esophagus occurred, with slow return to normal in the ensuing five minutes (Fig. 12.3). These observations indicate that chest

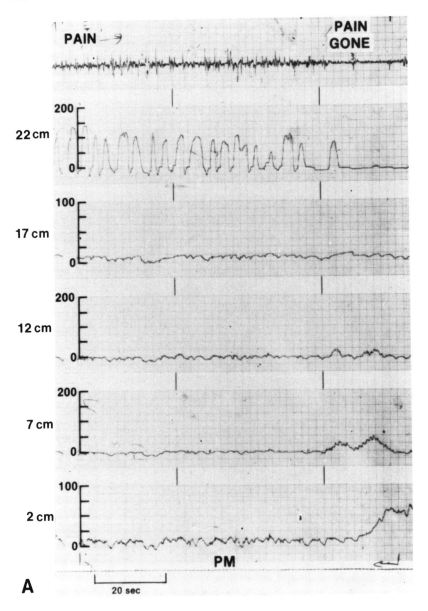

FIGURE 12.3 Esophageal pressure recordings during rapid ingestion of soft ice cream in a normal volunteer. Tracings from bottom to top are 2, 7, 12, 17, and 22 cm above the sphincter. Top trace is a swallow signal. Note complete absence of contractile activity in the distal esophagus during chest pain induced by the cold material **(A)**. Slow progressive return of distal peristalsis is seen as the esophagus is rewarmed with room-temperature water swallows (WS) at 20-sec intervals **(B)**.

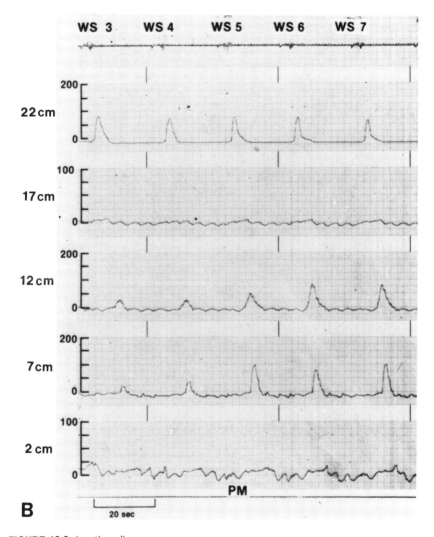

WS 3   WS 4   WS 5   WS 6   WS 7

22 cm

17 cm

12 cm

7 cm

2 cm

PM

B

20 sec

FIGURE 12.3 *(continued)*

pain induced by rapid ingestion of cold material is associated with esophageal smooth muscle that is relaxed and flaccid, rather than spastic.

Hot water, on the other hand, accelerates the response of the esophagus to a swallow.[18] This is reflected by increased speed of wave propagation and waves of shorter duration, with no change in peristaltic amplitude. Hot water does not alter normal progressive peristalsis.

REFERENCES

1. Stanciu C, Bennett JR: Smoking and gastroesophageal reflux. *Br Med J* 1972;3:793–795.
2. Chattopadhyay DK, Greaney ML, Irvin TT: Effect of cigarette smoking on the lower oesophageal sphincter. *Gut* 1977;18:833–835.
3. Dennish GW, Castell DO: Inhibitory effect of smoking on the lower esophageal sphincter. *N Engl J Med* 1971;284:1136–1137.
4. Rattan S, Goyal RK: Effect of nicotine on the lower oesophageal sphincter. *Gastroenterology* 1975;69:154–159.
5. McMahon TP, Castell JA, Castell DO: The effect of nicotine-containing products on the human esophagus (abstr). *Gastroenterology* 1986;90:1546A.
6. Kjelling G, Tibbling L: Influence of body position, dry and water swallows, smoking and alcohol on esophageal acid clearing. *Scand J Gastroenterol* 1978;13:283–288.
7. Hogan WJ, Viegas de Andrade SR, Winship DH: Ethanol-induced acute esophageal motor dysfunction. *J Appl Physiol* 1972;32:755–760.
8. Winship DH, Caflish CR, Zboralske FF, et al: Deterioration of esophageal peristalsis in patients with alcoholic neuropathy. *Gastroenterology* 1968;55:173–178.
9. Babka TC, Castell DO: On the genesis of heartburn. *Am J Dig Dis* 1973;18:391–397.
10. Nebel OT, Castell DO: Lower esophageal sphincter pressure changes after food ingestion. *Gastroenterology* 1972;63:778–783.
11. Sigmund CJ, McNally EF: The action of a carminative on the lower esophageal sphincter. *Gastroenterology* 1969;75:240–243.
12. Dennish GW, Castell DO: Caffeine and the lower esophageal sphincter. *Am J Dig Dis* 1972;17:991–993.
13. Cohen S, Booth GH: Gastric acid secretion and lower esophageal sphincter pressure in response to coffee and caffeine. *N Engl J Med* 1975;293:897–899.
14. Thomas FB, Steinbaugh JT, Fromkes JJ, et al: Inhibitory effect of coffee on lower esophageal sphincter pressure. *Gastroenterology* 1980;79:1262–1266.
15. Salmon PR, Fedail SS, Wurzner HP, et al: Effect of coffee on human lower esophageal dysfunction. *Digestion* 1981;21:69.
16. Price SF, Smithson KW, Castell DO: Food sensitivity in reflux esophagitis. *Gastroenterology* 1978;75:240–243.
17. Lloyd DA, Borda IT: Food induced heartburn: effect of osmolarity. *Gastroenterology* 1981:80:740–741.
18. Winship DH, Viegas de Andrade SR, Zboralske FF: Influence of bolus temperature on human esophagus motor function. *J Clin Invest* 1970;409:243–250.
19. Meyer GW, Castell DO: Human esophageal response during chest pain induced by swallowing cold liquids. *JAMA* 1981;246:2057–2059.

CHAPTER 13

Secondary Motility Disorders

Martin W. Scobey, MD

INTRODUCTION

In addition to the primary esophageal motility disorders that have been described in previous chapters, a variety of secondary esophageal motility problems may occur as a result of certain systemic conditions (Table 13.1). In general, esophageal manometry is most useful in evaluating those processes that are likely to produce lower esophageal dysfunction and may even be helpful in diagnosing certain diseases such as progressive systemic sclerosis[1] and chronic idiopathic intestinal pseudo-obstruction.[2] In the evaluation of oropharyngeal and upper esophageal dysfunction, cineradiography will usually yield more information. This is largely due to the technical difficulties encountered in assessing the oropharynx and upper esophagus by manometry, as well as a lack of reproducible normal manometric data in regard to this anatomical area.

TABLE 13.1 Conditions Associated with Secondary Esophageal Motor Dysfunction

Collagen-vascular diseases
Endocrine and metabolic disorders
Neuromuscular diseases
Chronic idiopathic intestinal pseudo-obstruction
Chagas' disease
Aging

163

COLLAGEN-VASCULAR DISEASES

The collagen-vascular diseases (Table 13.2) are comprised of a large group of acquired disorders of unknown cause, which characteristically exhibit multisystem involvement with immunologic and inflammatory changes in connective tissue. The esophagus may be affected by almost any of these diseases, although involvement (and therefore abnormal esophageal manometry) is most commonly seen with progressive systemic sclerosis (PSS), mixed connective tissue disease (MCTD), and polymyositis and dermatomyositis.

Progressive Systemic Sclerosis

PSS is a disease characterized by fibrosis and degenerative changes in the skin, synovium, and parenchyma of certain organs, notably the heart, kidneys, lungs, intestines, and esophagus.[3] General criteria for the diagnosis are established and may be found elsewhere.[4] Two forms of the generalized disease exist, PSS with diffuse scleroderma (a more fulminant form with early appearance of disease in various internal organs) and the CREST (calcinosis, Raynaud phenomenon, esophageal dysfunction, sclerodactyly, telangiectasia) syndrome.[3] Regardless of the form, the esophagus is involved in approximately 75% to 85% of all patients with PSS, by either manometric or radiographic criteria.[1,5,6]

The pathologic changes of PSS,[7] which are confined to the lower two-thirds (the smooth muscle portion) of the esophagus, give rise to a diminished to absent lower esophageal peristalsis and an incompetent lower esophageal sphincter (LES). Thus, the most common esophageal symptoms attributed to PSS are heartburn and regurgitation, which result from gastroesophageal (GE) reflux.[8,9]

TABLE 13.2 Collagen-Vascular Diseases

Progressive systemic sclerosis
Mixed connective tissue disease
Polymyositis and dermatomyositis
Systemic lupus erythematosis
Rheumatoid arthritis
Juvenile arthritis
Vasculitides
Sjögren's syndrome
Miscellaneous

The manometric features of PSS are quite distinctive and include low to absent LES pressure (LESP), weak to absent distal esophageal peristalsis, and normal upper esophageal peristalsis and sphincter pressure (Fig. 13.1).[8,9] Radiographically, distal esophageal distention with a patulous GE junction and hiatal hernia is often seen. Since this disorder predominantly affects the lower esophagus, manometry should be more useful in its evaluation, and in fact it has been shown to be more sensitive than radiography for detecting early esophageal involvement by PSS.[10] Occasionally, esophageal manometry may be quite valuable to help support a diagnosis of PSS in equivocal cases.

Mixed Connective Tissue Disease

This disorder represents a mixture of clinical features found in PSS, polymyositis, and systemic lupus erythematosus (SLE), and is noted for the presence of high titers of a circulating antibody for a nuclear ribonucleoprotein antigen.[11] More than 60% of all patients have esophageal involvement by either manometry or cineradiography.[12] The manometric findings are very similar to PSS, with a decrease in both LESP and distal esophageal peristalsis.

Polymyositis and Dermatomyositis

Polymyositis (termed dermatomyositis when accompanied by the classic skin eruption) is a diffuse inflammatory disease of striated muscle in which the patient exhibits symmetrical muscle weakness and atrophy of the proximal muscle groups.[13] Rigid criteria for the diagnosis of this disorder have not been established and, in fact, it may have overlapping clinical and laboratory features with other collagen-vascular diseases. The esophagus appears to be involved in approximately 60% to 70% of cases by radiographic or manometric standards.[14]

Since the upper one-third of the esophagus is primarily involved in this particular disease, esophageal symptoms relate to upper esophageal dysfunction, with aspiration, nasopharyngeal regurgitation, and oropharyngeal dysphagia being noted.[9,14] Some symptoms related to lower esophageal dysfunction have also been reported.[14]

The manometric and radiographic features of polymyositis are shown in Table 13.3.[1,14] It should again be emphasized that in this disorder, as opposed to PSS, radiography is the more useful tool for evaluation because of the prominent skeletal muscle involvement. The detection of lower esophageal abnormalities by manometry[14] may still reflect overlap between this disease and other collagen-vascular disorders.

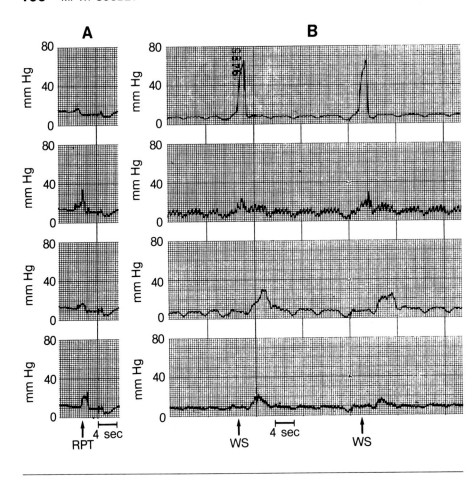

Other Collagen-Vascular Diseases

Esophageal symptoms are not common in SLE, although 25% to 35% of unselected patients will have abnormalities by manometry.[5,15] These findings appear to be a combination of the abnormalities seen in PSS and polymyositis, with decreased upper and lower esophageal peristalsis and LESP. Findings consistent with diffuse esophageal spasm have also been described in one report.[16]

Rheumatoid arthritis (RA), like SLE, does not usually produce major esophageal symptoms. Manometric abnormalities that have been reported are rather mild, with only a decrease in esophageal peristaltic amplitude being noted in 30% of patients in one study.[17]

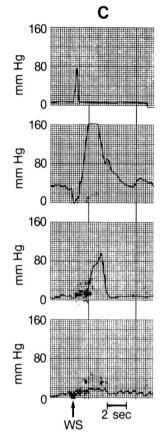

FIGURE 13.1 Esophageal motility tracing from a patient with PSS showing the classic manometric findings. **(A)** Low LES pressure seen during rapid pull-through (RPT) of the manometric catheter. Pressures were recorded at four sequential sites that were 1 cm apart, proximal (top) to distal (bottom). **(B)** Normal peristaltic amplitude in the proximal esophagus with decreased peristaltic amplitude distally after wet swallows (WS). Recording sites are at 18, 13, 8, and 3 cm from the LES (top to bottom). **(C)** Normal pharyngeal contraction and coordinated UES relaxation after a wet swallow (WS) demonstrated in top two tracings. Normal proximal esophageal peristaltic amplitude and decreased distal peristaltic amplitude are again demonstrated in bottom two tracings.

TABLE 13.3 Manometric and Radiographic Features of Polymyositis

Manometry
    Decreased UES pressure
    Decreased amplitude of pharyngeal contractions
    Decreased amplitude of proximal esophageal peristalsis
    (?) Decreased amplitude of lower esophageal peristalsis
    (?) Decreased LES pressure
Radiography
    Nasopharyngeal reflux
    Tracheal aspiration
    Disorganized pharyngeal emptying
    Vallecular pooling

The extent of esophageal dysfunction caused by other collagen vascular diseases is difficult to determine, due to the low incidence of these syndromes and the small numbers of patients studied. In primary Sjögren's syndrome, a disorder characterized by diminished lacrimal and salivary gland secretions, decreased upper esophageal peristalsis has been described in nine out of 10 patients in one investigation.[18] The exclusive use of dry swallows in that particular study, however, may have increased the frequency of the apparent abnormal swallows.[19] In another study, in which wet swallows were used for manometry, esophageal dysfunction was noted in 36% of 22 patients.[20] The pattern of dysfunction was not consistent, however. Different abnormalities observed included aperistalsis, triphasic tertiary contractions, nonperistaltic contractions, and low-amplitude contractions.

Bechet's syndrome, in which oral ulcers, genital ulcers, and iritis are noted, may also involve the esophagus with ulcers.[21,22] Manometry has not been systematically performed in patients with this particular disorder, and no specific motility pattern has been attributed to the disease.

ENDOCRINE AND METABOLIC DISORDERS
Diabetes Mellitus

It is fairly well established that esophageal manometric and radiographic abnormalities are common in diabetic patients with peripheral neuropathy.[23-31] The clinical significance of this fact is uncertain, however, since most of these patients are asymptomatic. The pathophysiology of these abnormalities is felt to be the degenerative effects of diabetes mellitus on the automatic nervous system, rather than smooth muscle dysfunction, as evidenced by histologic[32,33] and pharmacologic[28,29,31] data.

Manometric abnormalities were first described in detail in 1969 by Mandelstam et al.[24] They noted a decrease in the amplitude of peristalsis, a decrease in primary peristalsis, and a decrease in LESP in a small group of diabetics, all with autonomic neuropathy. These types of findings in diabetics with[28] and without[27] neuropathy were also noted by later investigators. In a larger study examining 50 diabetics with and without peripheral neuropathy, Hollis and co-workers[29] noted a decrease in primary peristalsis (greater than 10% absence of peristaltic response to a swallow), an increase in repetitive contractions (two or more contractions in greater than 25% of swallows), and an increase in spontaneous contractions (greater than 10 during a 35-min study), mainly in diabetics with peripheral neuropathy. No differences were noted in peristaltic amplitude or LES pressure in any of the groups, although there was a mild but significant decrease in peristaltic velocity in the diabetics with peripheral neuropathy.

More recently, Loo et al[31] have described another manometric abnormality in diabetics with peripheral neuropathy — an increased incidence of peristaltic double – peaked pressure complexes (Fig. 13.2A). The significance of this finding remains to be determined, since double-peaked waves do occur in normals (Fig. 13.2B) and the high incidence of double-peaked waves (> 95% of all peristaltic swallows) noted in their group of diabetics has not been confirmed in other diabetics studied with manometry.[34]

The different findings attributed to diabetes mellitus in the studies cited have not been explained, although they may in part be due to the development and use of better manometric equipment in later studies. Regardless, one can state that diabetics in general have a higher incidence of disordered esophageal peristalsis when compared to normals. This abnormal peristalsis may be manifest by minor findings such as occasional nontransmitted swallows and spontaneous activity (Fig. 13.3), or be so marked as to resemble diffuse spasm (Fig. 13.4).

Thyroid Disease

Although the literature is scant on this subject, esophageal motor abnormalities have been seen in either hyperthyroidism or hypothyroidism. An increase in the velocity of esophageal peristalsis has been described in one small group of patients with Graves' disease, which reverted to normal with treatment.[35] This abnormality did not appear to have any clinical significance in terms of producing symptoms, however. Diffuse esophageal spasm has also been described in one patient with thyrotoxic myopathy,[36] although this finding does not appear to be common. With myxedema, on the other hand, dysphagia is not an uncommon complaint and, in fact, a decrease in peristaltic amplitude, velocity, and primary peristalsis has been noted in one group of patients studied.[37] Another report has noted a decrease in LES pressure as well.[38] It appears that abnormalities revert to normal with treatment of the myxedema.[37,38] An additional abnormality of incomplete relaxation of the upper esophageal sphincter (UES) has also been described in one case report.[39] The mechanism of these esophageal abnormalities is unknown.

Amyloidosis

Manometric abnormalities that have been attributed to amyloidosis include a decrease in LES pressure, a decrease in both upper and lower esophageal peristaltic amplitude, simultaneous contractions, and even an achalasialike picture.[40,41] In the largest series reported, greater than 60% of patients with systemic amyloidosis had esophageal manometric abnormalities.[41] These derangements have been attributed to random deposition of amyloid in the

170

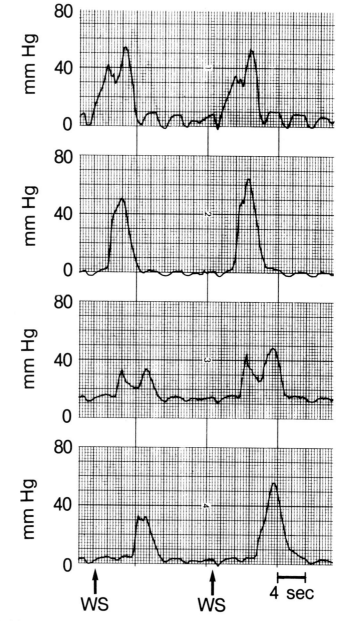

A

FIGURE 13.2 (A) Esophageal motility tracing from a diabetic patient showing frequent double-peaked peristaltic contractions after wet swallows (WS). Recordings are located at 18, 13, 8, and 3 cm above the LES (top to bottom). **(B)** In comparison, an esophageal motility tracing from a normal patient showing similar double-peaked peristaltic contractions.

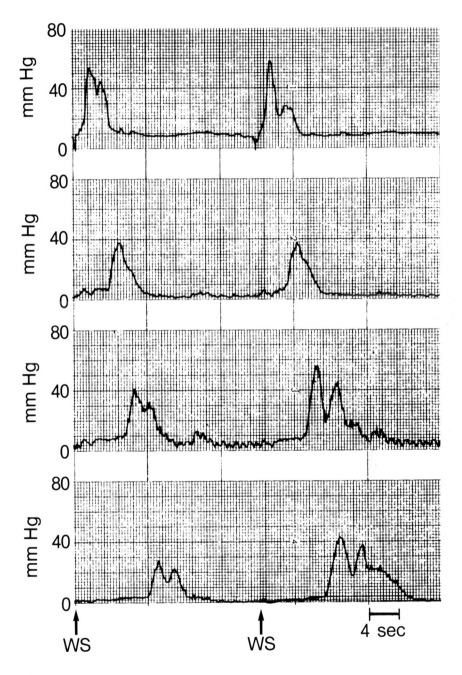

B

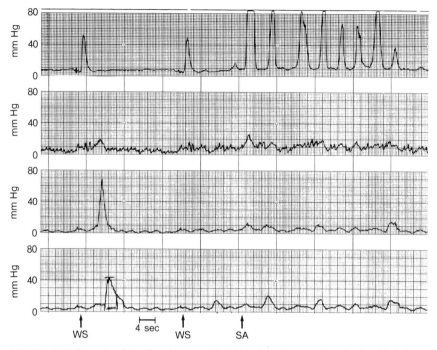

FIGURE 13.3 Example of the disordered peristalsis that may be seen in patients with diabetes mellitus. In this tracing there is a normal peristaltic response to the first wet swallow (WS), followed by a nontransmitted wave to the second wet swallow. Finally, spontaneous, repetitive activity (SA) is noted, some of which appears to be completely transmitted. Recordings are located at 18, 13, 8, and 3 cm above the LES (top to bottom).

muscle, and possibly the nerves, of the esophagus.[41,42] Similar manometric findings have also been noted in familial amyloid polyneuropathy.[43]

NEUROMUSCULAR DISORDERS

Esophageal motility may be affected by a number of neuromuscular problems. Unfortunately, most of the manometric data pertaining to these disorders has been accumulated from studies done in the 1960s using nonperfused manometric equipment and dry swallows. Since neuromuscular disorders generally tend to produce oropharyngeal and upper esophageal abnormalities,[44] the technical limitations of manometry in evaluating these

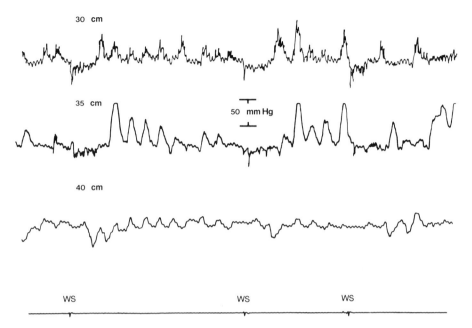

FIGURE 13.4 Esophageal motility tracing from a patient with diabetes mellitus exhibiting DES-like activity in response to wet swallows (WS). Recordings are located at 30, 35, and 40 cm from the nares (top to bottom).

disorders must also be considered. As one might expect, cineradiography has generally yielded more information in their evaluation.[45] Nevertheless, several neuromuscular disorders have been studied manometrically as summarized in the following sections.

Myotonic Dystrophy

This disorder is an autosomal-dominant familial disease that results in myotonia and distal muscle wasting and weakness. Esophageal manometric studies performed in patients with this disorder have shown both striated and smooth muscle involvement, as evidenced by a decrease in the UES pressure, and a decrease in the amplitude of contraction in the pharynx, upper esophagus, and lower esophagus.[36,46–48] Prolonged pharyngeal contraction has also been observed[46] (Fig. 13.5) and is probably evidence of the myotonia that is the hallmark of this disease. Dysphagia may be a frequent complaint in patients with this disorder.[36,46]

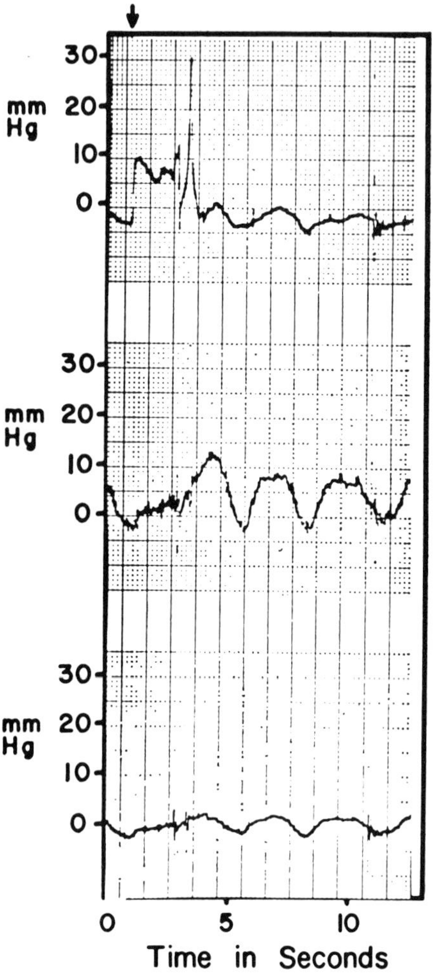

FIGURE 13.5 Tracing from a patient showing prolongation of pharyngeal contraction and decreased amplitude of contraction in the proximal and distal esophagus after a swallow (arrow). Recording sites are in the pharynx and mid- and distal esophagus (top to bottom). (From Harvey JC, Sherbourne DH, Siegel CI: Smooth muscle involvement in myotonic dystrophy. *Am J Med* 1965;339:81–90. Reprinted with permission.)

Myasthenia Gravis

Patients with myasthenia gravis have been shown to exhibit a decrease in the amplitude of peristaltic contractions mainly in the upper esophagus, the amount of decrease dependent upon how severely the particular patient is affected by the disease.[36] In some cases, this proximal esophageal weakness may only be apparent with repetitive swallows (Fig. 13.6).

Multiple Sclerosis

This problem may cause a variety of esophageal motility abnormalities, presumably due to the variable nervous system involvement by the disease process. Simultaneous peristaltic waves, uncoordinated repetitive waves, decreased upper and lower esophageal sphincter relaxation, and patterns consistent with diffuse esophageal spasm (DES) have all been described.[36,49]

Parkinson's Disease

Dysphagia does not appear to be a very common complaint in patients with Parkinson's disease, although esophageal abnormalities can frequently be

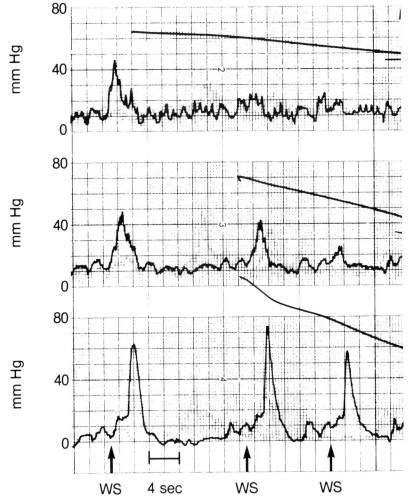

FIGURE 13.6 Esophageal motility tracing from a patient with myasthenia gravis showing a decrease in proximal esophageal peristaltic amplitude with repetitive wet swallows (WS). Recordings are located at 13, 8, and 3 cm above the LES (top to bottom).

shown radiographically[45] and manometrically.[36] Manometric findings have included a diminished to absent peristaltic wave, decreased primary peristalsis, and an increase in spontaneous waves.[36] How many of these findings were actually due to medications used to treat the disease has not been clarified.

Cerebrovascular Diseases

These processes may give rise to abnormal esophageal motility tracings, especially if bilateral pyramidal tract involvement has occurred. An increase in simultaneous peristaltic waves, changes in LES pressure (either elevated or decreased), decreased primary peristalsis, and DES-like pictures have all been noted.[36] Abnormal UES function, resulting in oropharyngeal dysphagia, is characteristic of posterior-inferior cerebellar artery syndrome.

Amyotrophic Lateral Sclerosis

Varied manometric abnormalities have been attributed to this entity in the small number of patients studied. The abnormalities noted have been a decrease in primary peristalsis, a decrease in upper esophageal peristaltic wave amplitude, a decrease in UES pressure and a DES-like picture.[36]

Central Nervous System Lymphoma

Dysphagia associated with lymphoma is usually due to direct esophageal involvement by the disease. However, lymphomatous involvement of the CNS without direct esophageal involvement has been shown by manometry to produce dysphagia and proximal esophageal dysfunction in one report.[50]

CHRONIC IDIOPATHIC INTESTINAL PSEUDO-OBSTRUCTION

Chronic idiopathic intestinal pseudo-obstruction (CIIP) is a syndrome characterized by intermittent symptoms and signs of intestinal obstruction without evidence for actual mechanical blockage. At present, the disorder can only be diagnosed in the absence of other systemic illnesses that are known to cause a similar picture and, in actuality, it probably represents many etiologies that remain to be defined. The pathophysiology of this syndrome has likewise remained elusive.[51-54]

Various motility abnormalities throughout the bowel have been described in this disorder, but one area that appears to be consistently abnormal is the esophagus. At least 85% of all patients with CIIP have abnormal esophageal manometry.[51,52] Manometry in this disorder was first described in detail by Schuffler and Pope.[2] Most patients exhibit aperistalsis (either simultaneous or absent waves; Fig. 13.7) and variable abnormalities in the LES — often decreased to absent LES relaxation. The manometric picture can be very similar to achalasia and, in fact, positive mecholyl tests have been reported in some patients.[2] However, most patients with CIIP do not exhibit dysphagia[51,52,55] and those that do apparently do not respond to the usual treatment for achalasia.[2]

Because of the high occurrence of manometric abnormalities in these patients, we use esophageal motility testing as a screening test. The finding of normal esophageal motility should essentially exclude this diagnosis.

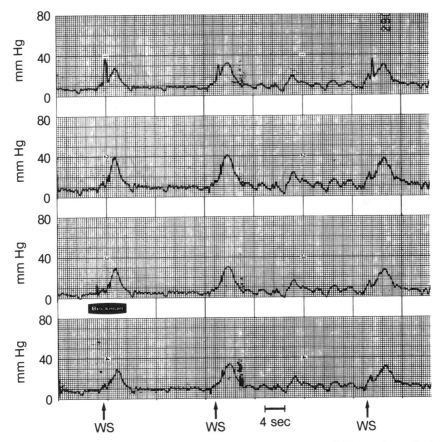

FIGURE 13.7 Simultaneous, nonperistaltic activity after wet swallows (WS), seen in a patient with CIIP. In this particular patient, the catheter tip could not be advanced past the LES. Recordings are located at 18, 13, 8, and 3 cm above the LES (top to bottom).

CHAGAS' DISEASE

Chagas' disease is caused by a protozoan, *Trypanosoma cruzi,* commonly found in South America. The disease affects multiple organs, including the myenteric plexus of the gastrointestinal tract, and produces esophageal manifestations identical to achalasia. Manometry, which may be abnormal even prior to symptoms, reveals a pattern indistinguishable from achalasia, with aperistalsis of the esophagus, spontaneous or repetitive waves, and delayed or incomplete relaxation of the LES.[56]

AGING AND THE ESOPHAGUS

Based upon radiographic[57] and manometric[58] studies performed in the early 1960s, it was initially felt that the aging process produced certain patterns of esophageal dysfunction. Further study of the aging esophagus with improved manometric techniques and the exclusion of systemic diseases known to cause esophageal motor abnormalities has, however, led to a reassessment of the effects of age on the esophagus.

The earliest manometric studies,[58] done with a small group of nonagenerians, demonstrated decreased primary peristalsis (defined as no contractions or simultaneous contractions of the esophagus in response to a swallow), decreased LES relaxation, and an increase in spontaneous contractions. However, patients with systemic diseases such as diabetes mellitus or other neurologic disorders were not necessarily excluded from that study. In addition, manometry was performed with nonperfused catheters and with the use of dry swallows, two factors that may have caused an underestimation of esophageal amplitude and an apparent decrease in primary peristalsis.

In 1974, Hollis and Castell[59] reported a study of 21 elderly men, 70 to 87 years old, with modern manometric equipment utilizing miniature intraesophageal transducers. (It is important to note that systemic diseases that may have affected esophageal function were excluded from this study.) They found only a mild decrease in the amplitude of esophageal peristaltic contractions with normal LES relaxation, primary peristalsis, velocity, and duration of contractions. Kahn et al[60] examined this problem a few years later, again excluding patients with systemic diseases. Their findings included a mild decrease in esophageal peristaltic amplitude, primary peristalsis, and LES relaxation with normal velocities. Finally, Csendes et al[61] studied esophageal manometry in a spectrum of normal asymptomatic adults from age 15 to 74. Peristaltic amplitude and duration, as well as LES pressure, showed no changes with age. There was, however, a slight decrease noted in the frequency of primary peristalsis.

Table 13.4 provides a summary of the findings related to age in the

TABLE 13.4 Manometric Studies on the Effects of Aging on the Esophagus[a]

Study	Year	Amplitude of Esophageal Peristalsis	Primary Peristalsis	LES Relaxation	Spontaneous Contractions	Duration of Peristaltic Waves
Soergel et al[58]	1964	N	↓↓	↓↓	↑↑	N
Hollis and Castell[59]	1974	→→	N→	N→	N	N
Khan et al[60]	1977	→	→→	→	NS	NS
Csendes et al[61]	1978	N	→	NS	NS	N

[a]N, normal; NS, not studied.

studies just discussed. Taken as a whole it would appear that the main effect of age on esophageal function is a mild decrease in the amplitude or force of esophageal contractions. There probably is also a mild decrease in the frequency of primary peristalsis, but not to the extent first described in the early 1960s. The importance of these mild aberrations in esophageal function attributed to aging lies mainly in their recognition when interpreting motility tracings in the elderly. Severe motility abnormalities, when encountered, are most often due to systemic disease rather than to the aging process.

REFERENCES

1. Turner R, Lipshutz W, Miller W, et al: Esophageal dysfunction in collagen disease. *Am J Med Sci* 1973;265:191–199.
2. Schuffler MD, Pope CE II: Esophageal motor dysfunction in idiopathic intestinal pseudoobstruction. *Gastroenterology* 1976;70:677–682.
3. LeRoy EC: Scleroderma (systemic sclerosis), in Kelly WN, Harris ED Jr, Ruddy S, et al (eds): *Textbook of Rheumatology.* Philadelphia, Saunders, 1985, pp 1183–1205.
4. Masi AT, Rodnan GP, Medsger TA Jr, et al: Preliminary criteria for the classification of systemic sclerosis. *Arthritis Rheum* 1980;23:581–590.
5. Stevens MB, Hookman P, Siegel CI, et al: Aperistalsis of the esophagus in patients with connective-tissue disorders and Raynaud's phenomenon. *N Engl J Med* 1964;270:1218–1222.
6. Clements PJ, Kadell B, Ippoliti A, et al: Esophageal motility in progressive systemic sclerosis (PSS). Comparison of cine-radiographic and manometric evaluation. *Dig Dis Sci* 1979;24:639–644.
7. D'Angelo WA, Fries JF, Masi AT, et al: Pathologic observations in systemic sclerosis (scleroderma). *Am J Med* 1969;46:428–440.
8. Cohen S, Laufer I, Snape WJ Jr, et al: The gastrointestinal manifestations of scleroderma; pathogenesis and management. *Gastroenterology* 1980;79:155–166.
9. Chobanian SJ, Castell DO: Esophageal abnormalities in systemic disease, in Castell DO, Johnson LF (eds): *Esophageal Function in Health and Disease.* New York, Elsevier Biomedical, 1983, pp 273–294.
10. Neschis M, Siegelman SS, Rotstein J, et al: The esophagus in progressive systemic sclerosis. A manometric and radiographic correlation. *Am J Dig Dis* 1970;15:443–446.
11. Sharp GC, Irvin WS, Tan EM, et al: Mixed connective tissue disease; an apparently distinct rheumatic disease syndrome associated with a specific antibody to an extractable nuclear antigen (ENA). *Am J Med* 1972;52:148–159.
12. Winn D, Gerhardt D, Winship D, et al: Esophageal function in steroid-treated patients with mixed connective tissue disease (MCTD) (abstr). *Clin Res* 1976;24:545A.
13. Bradley WG: Inflammatory diseases of muscle, in Kelley WN, Harris ED Jr, Ruddy S, et al (eds): *Textbook of Rheumatology.* Philadelphia, Saunders, 1985, pp 1225–1245.
14. Jacob H, Berkowitz D, McDonald E, et al: The esophageal motility disorder of polymyositis. A prospective study. *Arch Intern Med* 1983;143:2262–2264.
15. Ramiraz-Mata M, Reyes PA, Alarcon-Segovia D, et al: Esophageal motility in systemic lupus erythematosus. *Am J Dig Dis* 1974;19:132–136.
16. Peppercorn MA, Docken WP, Rosenberg S: Esophageal motor dysfunction in systemic lupus erythematosus. Two cases with unusual features. *JAMA* 1979;242:1895–1896.

17. Sun DCH, Roth SH, Mitchell CS, et al: Upper gastrointestinal disease in rheumatoid arthritis. *Am J Dig Dis* 1974;19:405–410.
18. Ramirez-Mata M, Pena-Ancira FF, Alarcon-Segovia D: Abnormal esophageal motility in primary Sjögren's syndrome. *J Rheumatol* 1976;3:63–69.
19. Richter JE, Wu WC, Johns DN, et al: Esophageal manometry in 95 healthy adult volunteers: variability of pressure with age and frequency of abnormal contractions. *Dig Dis Sci* (in press).
20. Tsianos EB, Chiras CD, Drosos AA, et al: Oesophageal dysfunction in patients with primary Sjögren's syndrome. *Ann Rheum Dis* 1985;44:610–613.
21. Brodie TE, Ochsner JL: Behcet's syndrome with ulcerative oesophagitis: report of the first case. *Thorax* 1973;28:637–640.
22. Levack B, Hanson D: Behcet's disease of the oesophagus. *J Laryngol Otol* 1979;93:99–101.
23. Mandelstam P, Lieber A: Esophageal dysfunction in diabetic neuropathy-gastroenteropathy. *JAMA* 1967;201:88–92.
24. Mandelstam P, Siegel CI, Lieber A, et al: The swallowing disorder in patients with diabetic neuropathy-gastroenteropathy. *Gastroenterology* 1969;56:1–12.
25. Silber W: Diabetes and oesophageal dysfunction. *Br Med J* 1969;3:688–690.
26. Vix VA: Esophageal motility in diabetes mellitus. *Radiology* 1969;92:363–364.
27. Vela AR, Balart LA: Esophageal motor manifestations in diabetes mellitus. *Am J Surg* 1970;119:21–26.
28. Stewart IM, Hosking DJ, Preston BJ, et al: Oesophageal motor changes in diabetes mellitus. *Thorax* 1976;31:278–283.
29. Hollis JB, Castell DO, Braddom RL: Esophageal function in diabetes mellitus and its relation to peripheral neuropathy. *Gastroenterology* 1977;73:1098–1102.
30. Russell COH, Gannan R, Coatsworth J, et al: Relationship among esophageal dysfunction, diabetic gastroenteropathy and peripheral neuropathy. *Dig Dis Sci* 1983;28:289–293.
31. Loo FD, Dodds WJ, Soergel KH, et al: Multipeaked esophageal peristaltic pressure waves in patients with diabetic neuropathy. *Gastroenterology* 1985;88:485–491.
32. Smith B: Neuropathology of the oesophagus in diabetes mellitus. *J Neurol Neurosurg Psychiatry* 1974;37:1151–1154.
33. Rundles RW: Diabetic neuropathy. General review with report of 125 cases. *Medicine* 1945;24:111–151.
34. Richter JE, Wu WC, Castell DO: Double-peaked contraction waves—a variant of normal. *Gastroenterology* 1985;89:479–480.
35. Meshkinpour H, Afrasiabi MA, Valenta LJ: Esophageal motor function in Graves' disease. *Dig Dis Sci* 1979;24:159–161.
36. Fischer RA, Ellison GW, Thayer WR, et al: Esophageal motility in neuromuscular disorders. *Ann Intern Med* 1965;63:229–248.
37. Christensen J: Esophageal manometry in myxedema. *Gastroenterology* 1967;52:1130.
38. Eastwood GL, Braverman LE, White EM, et al: Reversal of lower esophageal sphincter hypotension and esophageal aperistalsis after treatment for hypothyroidism. *J Clin Gastroenterol* 1982;4:307–310.
39. Wright RA, Penner DB: Myxedema and upper esophageal dysmotility. *Dig Dis Sci* 1981;26:376–377.
40. Gilat T, Spiro HM: Amyloidosis and the gut. *Am J Dig Dis* 1968;13:619–633.
41. Rubinow A, Burakoff R, Cohen AS, et al: Esophageal manometry in systemic amyloidosis. A study of 30 patients. *Am J Med* 1983;75:951–956.
42. Liske E, Chou S, Thompson HG: Peripheral and autonomic neuropathy in amyloidosis. *JAMA* 1963;186:432–434.
43. Burakoff R, Rubinow A, Cohen AS: Esophageal manometry in familial amyloid polyneuropathy. *Am J Med* 1985;79:85–89.

44. Mukhopadhyay A, Graham DY: Esophageal motor dysfunction in systemic diseases. *Arch Intern Med* 1976;136:583–588.

45. Silbiger ML, Pikielney R, Donner MW: Neuromuscular disorders affecting the pharynx. Cineradiographic analysis. *Invest Radiol* 1967;2:442–448.

46. Harvey JC, Sherbourne DH, Siegel CI: Smooth muscle involvement in myotonic dystrophy. *Am J Med* 1965;39:81–90.

47. Pierce JW, Creamer B, MacDermot V: Pharynx and oesophagus is dystrophia myotonica. *Gut* 1965;6:392–395.

48. Siegel CI, Hendrix TR, Harvey JC: The swallowing disorder in myotonia dystrophica. *Gastroenterology* 1966;50:541–550.

49. Daly DD, Code CF, Andersen HA: Disturbances of swallowing and esophageal motility in patients with multiple sclerosis. *Neurology* 1962;12:250–256.

50. Benjamin SB, Eisold J, Gerhardt DC, et al: Central nervous system lymphoma presenting as dysphagia. *Dig Dis Sci* 1982;27:155–160.

51. Hanks JB, Meyers WC, Andersen DK, et al: Chronic primary intestinal pseudo-obstruction. *Surgery* 1981;89:175–182.

52. Schuffler MD, Rohrmann CA, Chaffe RG, et al: Chronic intestinal pseudo-obstruction. A report of 27 cases and review of the literature. *Medicine* 1981;60:173–196.

53. Sullivan MA, Snape WJ Jr, Matarazzo SA, et al: Gastrointestinal myoelectrical activity in idiopathic intestinal pseudo-obstruction. *N Engl J Med* 1977;297:233–238.

54. Sarna SK, Daniel EE, Waterfall WE, et al: Postoperative gastrointestinal electrical and mechanical activities in a patient with idiopathic intestinal pseudoobstruction. *Gastroenterology* 1978;74:112–120.

55. Schuffler MD: Chronic intestinal pseudo-obstruction syndromes. *Med Clin North Am* 1981;65:1331–1358.

56. Bettarello A, Pinotti HW: Oesophageal involvement in Chagas' disease. *Clin Gastroenterol* 1976;5:103–117.

57. Zboralske FF, Amberg JR, Soergel KH: Presbyesophagus: cineradiographic manifestations. *Radiology* 1964;82:463–467.

58. Soergel KH, Zboralske FF, Amberg JR: Presbyesophagus: esophageal motility in nonagerians. *J Clin Invest* 1964;43:1472–1479.

59. Hollis JB, Castell DO: Esophageal function in elderly men. A new look at "presbyesophagus." *Ann Intern Med* 1974;80:371–374.

60. Khan TA, Shragge BW, Crispin JS, et al: Esophageal motility in the elderly. *Am J Dig Dis* 1977;22:1049–1054.

61. Csendes A, Guiraldes E, Bancalari A, et al: Relation of gastroesophageal sphincter pressure and esophageal contractile waves to age in man. *Scand J Gastroenterol* 1978;13:443–447.

CHAPTER 14

The Upper Esophageal Sphincter

W. E. Roger Green, MB, FRCS (England), MS (London)
and Donald O. Castell, MD, FACP

The term upper esophageal sphincter (UES) is a definition given to a zone of intraluminal high pressure that exists between the pharynx and esophagus. This high-pressure zone (HPZ), as determined by manometry, may be 2.5 – 4.5 cm in length. There is general agreement that the cricopharyngeal muscle forms at least part of this HPZ but, since this muscle is only 1 – 2 cm wide, it is likely that some of the HPZ is made up by the muscles of the hypopharynx, the esophagus, or both.[1] The UES is closed at rest and opens momentarily in response to a swallow. Electromyographic evidence from studies in the opossum has shown that both the cricopharyngeal and inferior pharyngeal constrictor muscles behave functionally as the UES, being tonically contracted at rest and inhibited and relaxed during swallowing.[2] The evidence available in humans, however, favors the cricopharyngeus as the only part of the HPZ to display a tonic contraction-relaxation pattern typical of a sphincter muscle.[3,4] At the present time, the precise anatomical identity of the UES is undefined. There is, however, little doubt that while an HPZ of considerable length may be demonstrated by manometry, the maximum pressures recorded, which are the pressures of interest in clinical practice, are invariably confined to a 1- to 2-cm length between the hypopharynx and esophagus. It is this localized zone of maximum pressure that we refer to when the term UES is used in this chapter.

UPPER ESOPHAGEAL SPHINCTER PRESSURES

It has been difficult, for many reasons, to define a range of normal values for resting UES pressure. The fidelity of the recording system, the location and orientation of the pressure-sensitive device within the HPZ, the size and shape of the catheter assembly, and the rapidity with which it is moved through the sphincter have all been shown to have some effect upon the resulting UES pressure measurement. Recent improvements in intraluminal recording techniques have resulted in low-compliance systems, which can record rapid pressure changes that exceed 400 mm Hg/sec.[5] Careful attention to the orientation of the recording device within the sphincter has also been an important factor in obtaining reproducible pressure recordings from the UES. Radial asymmetry has been demonstrated by the use of multi-lumen catheters in which the direction of each side hole was known.[6,7] Within the UES, pressures recorded in the anterior and posterior directions exceed pressures recorded laterally by two or three times. Axial, or longitudinal, asymmetry has been identified by pull-through studies of the entire HPZ, again using catheters where the orientation of the recording orifices was known.[8] The highest anterior pressures in the UES are recorded near the pharynx, while the highest posterior pressures occur closer to the esophagus.

Two other factors may affect UES pressure recordings. It has been our experience[9] and that of others[10] that rapid pull-through (RPT) of the recording device through the UES yields higher pressures (by 25%–30%) than does a slow station pull-through (SPT). As a perfused catheter system is withdrawn slowly through the UES, the infusion of water into the hypopharynx may increase UES pressure, and eventually induce the patient to swallow. Both these effects appear to be a mechanical stimulation of the UES and cause it to contract beyond its usual resting-pressure level. The reported values for UES pressure in normal subjects encompass such a wide range that no single normal value emerges from any of the studies (Table 14.1). The range of maximum and minimum UES pressures recorded from 20 normal volunteers in our laboratory, using a low-compliance system and an SPT of an oval and round catheter, is shown in Figure 14.1.

THE HYPOPHARYNX

The muscles of the pharynx contract during swallowing in an orderly sequence and create a propulsive wave that sweeps the bolus into the esophagus through the relaxed and open UES. The pharyngeal pressure complex

TABLE 14.1 Resting Upper Esophageal Sphincter Pressure in Normal Subjects[a]

Reference	Year	Number Studied	Maximum (mm Hg)	Minimum (mm Hg)
Winans[6]	1972	18	101	32
Berlin et al[7]	1977	6	81	46
Welch et al[8]	1979	13	136	50
Gerhardt et al[11]	1980	20	101	48
Hellmans et al[10]	1981	10	115	30
Knuff et al[12]	1982	15	92	42
Green[b]	1986	20	64	29

[a]All studies were station pull throughs, using low-compliance perfused catheter system with known orientation of the side openings.
[b]See Figure 14.1.

increases in amplitude and decreases in duration as it approaches the UES. Maximal pharyngeal pressures are generated just proximal to the UES, in the anatomical hypopharynx. From a functional point of view, therefore, the muscles of the hypopharynx behave as a propulsive unit. These high pressures may average 130 mm Hg, and have been reported to be as high as 600 mm Hg.[13] They are of short duration, 0.5 sec or less,[13,14] and show rates of change in pressure that may exceed 500 mm Hg/sec. Because of the slower response rate of simple perfusion systems and the undesirable effects of the infused water in the hypopharynx, it is likely that solid-state intraluminal transducers will in the future replace the manometry catheter for accurate quantitation of pharyngeal pressures.[13,14]

Unlike the UES, the pressure profile within the lumen of the hypopharynx is symmetrical and, unlike the esophagus, the response to wet or dry swallows is the same.[13]

COORDINATION OF HYPOPHARYNX AND THE UPPER ESOPHAGEAL SPHINCTER

The coordination of events at the pharyngoesophageal junction is such that UES pressure falls at the time a swallow is initiated and this relaxation is maintained until the bolus, advancing ahead of the pharyngeal wave, has passed into the esophagus. Pharyngeal pressures measured 10 and 5 cm above the UES appear as a propagated wave that occurs in the middle of the

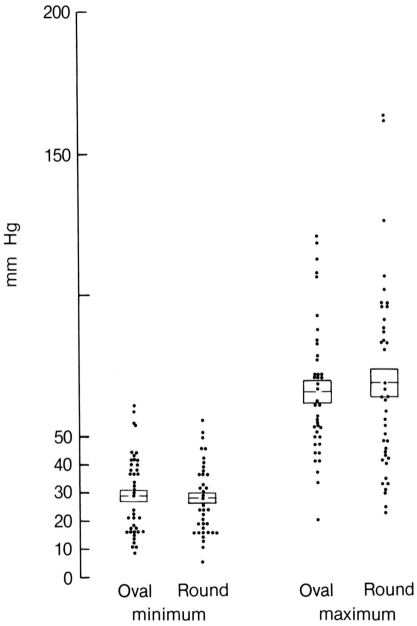

FIGURE 14.1 Upper esophageal sphincter resting pressures measured in 20 asymptomatic subjects, ages 19–65 years, by SPT of oval and round manometry catheters with radial side holes at 90°. Means ± 1 SE are shown by the boxes.

UES relaxation period (Fig. 14.2). As the hypopharyngeal pressure is sampled closer to the UES, the peak will occur closer to the end of the relaxation period until the pharyngeal stripping wave finally continues into the esophagus as the post-relaxation contraction of the UES itself (Fig. 14.3).

The normal events in the hypopharynx and UES have been studied in only two groups of normal subjects.[12,14] The manometric relationship is

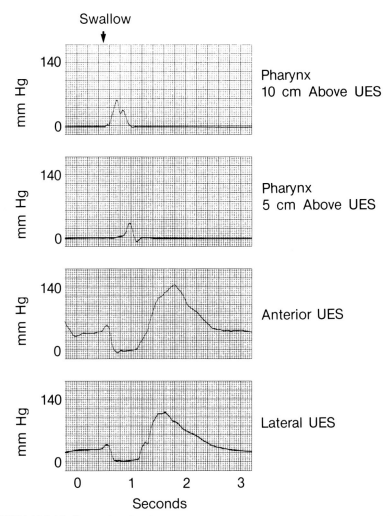

FIGURE 14.2 Motility tracing showing the coordinated sequence of pharyngeal contraction and UES relaxation. Two openings located 10 and 5 cm above the UES show aboral progression of the pharyngeal wave.

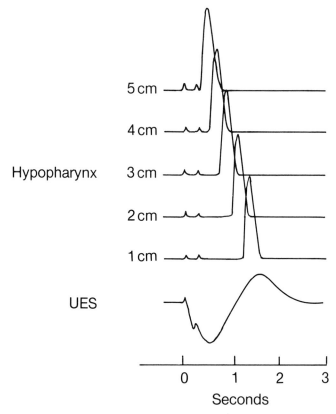

FIGURE 14.3 Relationship of hypopharyngeal contraction to UES relaxation. The propagated wave occurs in the middle of UES relaxation when measured 4–5 cm above the UES, but towards the end of the relaxation period if sampled only 1–2 cm above the sphincter.

shown in Figure 14.4 and the temporal relationship of events is shown in Table 14.2. More studies are required to establish a normal value for the duration of UES relaxation and the exact relationship of the pharyngeal contraction to this period. However, the basic principles of pharyngoesophageal coordination have been established by these two studies. If the pharyngeal wave, as measured 5 cm above the UES, does not occur during the middle one-third of the relaxation period it is then either misplaced or the UES relaxation itself is abnormal. If UES relaxation is prolonged, there is the potential for esophopharyngeal reflux; if it is attenuated the UES then may create an obstruction and cause dysphagia.

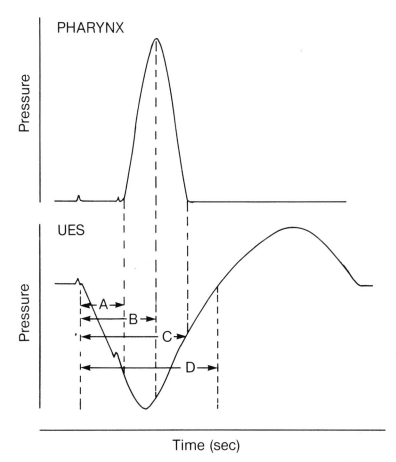

FIGURE 14.4 The graphic relationship between pharyngeal contraction and UES relaxation is based upon the data of Roed-Petersen[14] and Knuff et al.[12] Pressure and time units specified as A, B, and C define the position of the pharyngeal pressure wave within the period of UES relaxation (D). At maximum relaxation UES pressure approximates to intraesophageal pressure.

Three events are important in the recognition and definition of normal pharyngoesophageal function:

1. The pressure generated by the pharyngeal contraction wave
2. The resting tone of the UES, and its capacity to relax
3. The proper temporal relationship between 1 and 2

All three should be evaluated if pharyngoesophageal manometry is to be properly performed.

TABLE 14.2 Temporal Relationship Between Pharyngeal Contraction and UES Relaxation[a]

	Time (sec; 1 ± SE)			
	A	**B**	**C**	**D**
Roed-Petersen[14]	0.24 (0.05)	0.45	0.65	0.8 (0.02)
Knuff et al[12]	0.58 (0.05)	0.98 (0.06)	1.26 (0.07)	1.58 (0.07)

[a]The graphic relationship (see Fig. 14.4) between pharyngeal contraction and UES relaxation is based upon the data of Roed-Petersen[14] and Knuff et al.[12] Pressure and time units specified as A, B, and C define the position of the pharyngeal pressure wave within the period of UES relaxation (D). At maximum relaxation, UES pressure approximates intraesophageal pressure.

MANOMETRY OF THE PHARYNGOESOPHAGEAL JUNCTION

Because of the anatomical configuration of the UES, there has been considerable discussion concerning catheter shape and how to insure proper orientation within the sphincter. A catheter of oval configuration has been shown to regularly conform to the transverse orientation of the closed UES and, therefore, to allow the detection of the maximum (anterior-posterior) and minimum (lateral) pressures in this sphincter. Although this is true, the routine use of an oval catheter during standard esophageal manometry has not become popular because standard catheters for lower esophageal sphincter (LES) and esophageal body recordings have a round shape. Thus, we are often faced with the dilemma of either passing two catheters (one round and one oval) or developing oval catheters for use in the more distal esophagus. Recent studies in our laboratory have indicated that this problem can be reasonably circumvented by the use of a round catheter with at least four openings having angles not greater than 90° between each opening. In a comparison of a round catheter of this type with an oval catheter of the same diameter, identical pressures were obtained for maximum and minimum pressures of the four openings in the UES. These data are represented in Figure 14.1, and indicate that it is quite acceptable to use a standard round catheter for the entire study of the esophagus. A pull-through study of the UES, using such a catheter, is shown in Figure 14.5. At present, we use the 8-lumen catheter described in Chapter 3, using the four openings, arranged radially at 90° angles and spaced at 1-cm distances, to sequentially measure the UES pressures and to evaluate the pharyngeal-UES coordination.

Alternative methods of recording pharyngoesophageal pressures include the use of solid state probes in the pharynx and the Dent sleeve in place of the radial side holes in the UES. The sleeve may be of particular value if long-term recordings from the UES are planned, as it eliminates the problem of artifact caused by catheter movement within the sphincter and by sphincter movement over the catheter.[15] Neither of these alternatives has a place in routine manometry of the UES at the present time.

In studying the coordination of hypopharyngeal and UES motility, it has proven helpful to imprint on the record the time at which a swallow is initiated. A surface electrode, placed bilaterally over the geniohyoid muscles for electromyographic registration, is suitable for this purpose.

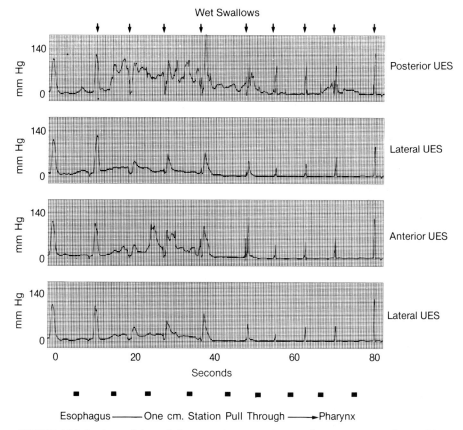

FIGURE 14.5 Station pull-through from esophagus to pharynx of a manometry catheter with four side holes at the same level, oriented at 90°. Wet swallows (arrows) were given after each 1-cm withdrawal. Baseline UES pressures recorded by the posterior and anterior openings are seen to be higher than pressures recorded laterally.

PROTOCOL FOR UPPER ESOPHAGEAL SPHINCTER MANOMETRY

1. Position the catheter in upper esophagus just below UES.
2. Initiate perfusion of UES side holes.
3. Establish baseline intraesophageal pressure
4. Determine UES resting pressures by 0.5-cm station pull-through with each of four orifices positioned at 90° angles.
5. Initiate perfusion of pharyngeal side hole.
6. Record hypopharyngeal-UES activity during 5–10 swallows, with one orifice in UES and one orifice 5 cm more proximal

ANALYSIS OF THE MANOMETRY RECORD

Abstraction of all of the following data from the record may not be of immediate relevance, but it will help develop a better understanding of normal and abnormal events associated with swallowing disorders.

1. Intraesophageal baseline pressure
2. Maximum, minimum, and mean UES resting pressure
3. Onset of UES relaxation (after swallow registration by EMG)
4. Residual pressure at low point of UES relaxation (calculate % UES relaxation)
5. Duration of UES relaxation
6. Duration and pressure of UES post-relaxation contraction
7. Peak hypopharyngeal pressure
8. Duration of hypopharyngeal wave
9. Position of hypopharyngeal wave within period of UES relaxation

   Coordinated
   Uncoordinated

10. Percent of swallows with coordinated pharyngoesophageal motility

ASSESSMENT OF UPPER ESOPHAGEAL SPHINCTER MANOMETRY DATA

A limited understanding of the mechanisms involved in oropharyngeal dysphagia, and a paucity of manometric data from the pharynx and UES in both normal and abnormal states, make it difficult to establish guidelines upon which to base an assessment of the record.

1. UES resting pressure is maximal in the anterior and posterior aspects of the sphincter and minimal in the lateral directions. The range of both within a group of normal subjects is wide. There is no current definition of the normal, hypertensive, or hypotensive UES. The functional significance of maximum, minimum, or mean UES pressure has not been established.

2. Relaxation of the UES begins with the reflex phase of swallowing. UES pressure falls to intraesophageal pressure $\pm$ 5 mm Hg. Resting pressure is reestablished within 0.8 – 1.6 sec.

3. UES contraction above resting baseline follows relaxation. Pressures generated in this phase persist for 1.5 – 2 sec. Normal values have not been established.

4. Contraction of the hypopharynx will be completed within the period of UES relaxation in 95% of swallows in normal subjects. However, even in disordered states, not every swallow may show incoordination, so a number of swallows must be performed to ensure that abnormality is detected.

5. No normal values for pressure or duration of the contraction wave have been established for the hypopharynx.

DISORDERS OF THE UPPER ESOPHAGEAL SPHINCTER

Swallowing difficulties are not uncommon and may represent a major cause of disability in the elderly.[16] Oropharyngeal dysphagia is a symptom, for which there are many causes, of disorder in a complex mechanism (Table 14.3). Abnormal function of the UES has been described in some of these conditions[17,18,19] but case reports have been few in number and the manometric data upon which the definition of abnormality has been based were all too often derived by methods now considered to be obsolete and invalid. Some aspects of UES dysfunction were also assigned only on the basis of radiological observations and there is a need today for these to be validated with current manometric techniques.

Abnormal UES function has been associated with dysphagia, particularly for liquids,[18] esophagopharyngeal regurgitation,[11] and globus sensation.[20] The disorder may be one of altered resting tone, or abnormal relaxation (Table 14.4).

Hypertensive Upper Esophageal Sphincter

High UES pressures have been described in so-called "spasm" of the cricopharyngeus and in globus sensation. Some authors have described higher

TABLE 14.3 Causes of Oropharyngeal Dysphagia: Neuromuscular Diseases

Central nervous system
  Cerebrovascular accident: bulbar or pseudobulbar palsy
  Parkinson disease
  Multiple sclerosis
  Amyotrophic lateral sclerosis
  Syringo-bulbia
  Stiff-man syndrome
  Brain stem tumor
  Tabes dorsalis
  Bulbar poliomyelitis
  Congenital Riley-Day syndrome (familial dysautonomia)
Peripheral nervous system
  Mononeuritis multiplex
  Diabetic neuropathy
  Miscellaneous neuropathies (diphtheria, tetanus, botulism)
Motor endplate
  Myasthenia gravis
Muscle
  Dystrophia myotonica
  Oculopharyngeal muscular dystrophy
  Polymyositis and dermatomyositis
  Metabolic myopathies (caused by thyrotoxemia, myxedema, steroids)

than normal pressures in the presence of esophagitis in patients with hiatus hernia and reflux.[21,22] Recent studies using current manometric techniques have shown that the UES resting pressure increases significantly in response to both saline and acid perfusion of the esophagus.[23] Patients with hiatus hernia have cervical symptoms, including pain and dysphagia.[24] Globus sensation has been associated with significantly higher-than-normal resting pressures[20] and there has been no more recent study to confirm or refute this observation.

TABLE 14.4 Causes of Oropharyngeal Dysphagia: Proposed Motility Disorders of the Upper Esophageal Sphincter

Hypertensive UES
Hypotensive UES
Abnormal UES relaxation
  Incomplete relaxation (achalasia)
  Delayed relaxation
  Premature closure

Hypotensive Upper Esophageal Sphincter

Lower-than-normal UES pressures have been reported in patients with esophagopharyngeal reflux.[11] Many of these patients had suffered from heartburn, and not only was UES pressure low, but the sphincter appeared to have lost the ability to increase pressure in response to intraesophageal acid. In this situation, UES hypotension may be secondary to esophageal damage with interruption of a protective reflex mechanism. UES hypotension is found after cricopharyngeal myotomy and after laryngectomy, yet these patients do not necessarily suffer from esophagopharyngeal reflux. Hypotension may also occur secondary to some neuromuscular disorders, including amyotrophic lateral sclerosis, myasthenia gravis, oculopharyngeal muscular dystrophy, and dystrophia myotonica.[17]

Abnormalities of Upper Esophageal Sphincter Relaxation

Three types of abnormality in UES relaxation have been described: incomplete relaxation, delayed relaxation, and premature closure.[25] The term "cricopharyngeal achalasia" has been used to refer to all of these abnormalities, but is perhaps better reserved specifically for the disorder of incomplete relaxation.

Incomplete Upper Esophageal Sphincter Relaxation (Cricopharyngeal Achalasia)

UES resting pressure normally falls to within 5 mm Hg of intraesophageal pressure, as a swallow is initiated, and does not return to baseline resting pressure until the bolus has passed, usually after a time interval of 0.8–1.6 sec. Patients with cricopharyngeal achalasia should show incomplete UES relaxation after the majority of swallows.[26] Achalasia has been described as an isolated phenomenon in children[27,28] and in adults, usually secondary to underlying disease, which may include cerebrovascular accident affecting the brain stem, bulbar poliomyelitis, stiff-man syndrome, thyrotoxic myopathy, and oculopharyngeal muscular dystrophy, and sometimes after pharyngectomy and laryngectomy.[10,17] A review of adult patients with cricopharyngeal achalasia reveals that this is primarily a problem of the elderly.[28] Although radiography may shown functional delay of barium at the level of the cricopharyngeus, the correlation with manometric studies showing incomplete relaxation is poor.[26] Neither study is ideal if used as the only investigation.

Delayed Upper Esophageal Sphincter Relaxation

Patients with familial dysautonomia (Riley-Day syndrome) may develop a number of disturbances related to autonomic function, including sucking and swallowing difficulty, which is usually present from birth.[29] Radiological studies have shown delayed opening of the cricopharyngeus[30] with normal pharyngeal motor activity. No manometric evidence for incoordination of this type has been reported.

Premature Upper Esophageal Sphincter Closure

It has been suggested that premature closure of the UES is an important factor in the pathogenesis of Zenker's diverticulum.[31] Manometric studies have not resolved this issue so far, since groups of patients have been reported where all,[31] some,[32] and none[12] showed premature UES closure. There has been general agreement that UES resting pressure is, if anything, lower than normal. While premature closure appears to be a condition that can occasionally be identified by manometry, no explanation for its occurrence has yet been proposed. True early closure of the UES implies a failure of the central inhibition of cricopharyngeal tone. However, local factors, including pharyngeal contraction and laryngeal elevation, may also affect the duration of UES relaxation. The universal acceptance of cricopharyngeal myotomy in the management of this condition has little justification, based upon the manometric data available today.

REFERENCES

1. Goyal RK, Cobb BW: Motility of the pharynx, esophagus, and esophageal sphincters, in Johnson LR (ed): *Physiology of the Gastrointestinal Tract*. New York, Raven Press, 1981, pp 359–391.
2. Asoh R, Goyal RK: Manometry and electromyography of the upper esophageal sphincter in the opossum. *Gastroenterology* 1978;74:514–520.
3. Shipp T, Deatsch WW, Robertson K: Pharyngoesophageal muscle activity during swallowing in man. *Laryngoscope* 1970;80:1–16.
4. Van-Overbeek JJM, Wit HP, Paping RHL, et al: Simultaneous manometry and electromyography in the pharyngoesophageal segment. *Laryngoscope* 1985;95:582–584.
5. Andorfer RC, Stef JJ, Dodds WJ, et al: Improved infusion system for intraluminal esophageal manometry. *Gastroenterology* 1977;73:23–27.
6. Winans CS: The pharyngoesophageal closure mechanism. A manometric study. *Gastroenterology* 1972;63:768–777.
7. Berlin BP, Fierstein JT, Tedesco F, et al: Manometric studies of the upper esophageal sphincter. *Ann Otol Rhinol Laryngol* 1977;86:598–602.
8. Welch RW, Luckmann K, Ricks PM, et al: Manometry of the normal upper esophageal sphincter and its alteration in laryngectomy. *J Clin Invest* 1979;63:1036–1041.
9. Green W, Castell J, Castell D: Comparison of oval and round catheters for manometric studies of upper esophageal sphincter (UES) pressure in man. *Gastroenterology* 1986;91:1054.
10. Hellmans J, Agg HO, Pelemans W, et al: Pharyngoesophageal swallowing disorders and the pharyngoesophageal sphincter. *Med Clin North Am* 1981;65:1149–1170.

11. Gerhardt DC, Castell DO, Winship DH, et al: Esophageal dysfunction in esophagopharyngeal regurgitation. *Gastroenterology* 1980;78:893–897.
12. Knuff TE, Benjamin SB, Castell DO: Pharyngoesophageal (Zenker's) diverticulum; a reappraisal. *Gastroenterology* 1982;82:734–736.
13. Dodds WJ, Hogan WJ, Lydon SB, et al: Quantitation of pharyngeal motor function in normal human subjects. *J Appl Physiol* 1975;39:692–696.
14. Roed-Peterson K: Manometric investigation of the pharyngoesophageal sphincter. *Dan Med Bull* 1979;26:282–287.
15. Dent J: A new technique for continuous sphincter pressure measurement. *Gastroenterology* 1976;71:263–267.
16. Donner MJ: Dysphagia editorial. *Dysphagia* 1986;1:1–2.
17. Vantrappen G, Hellmans J: *Diseases of the Esophagus*. New York, Springer-Verlag, 1974, pp 399–421.
18. Palmer ED: Disorders of the cricopharyngeus muscle; a review. *Gastroenterology* 1976;71:510–519.
19. Gerhardt DC, Winship DH. Cricopharyngeal disorders, in Cohen S, Soloway RD (eds): *Diseases of the Esophagus*. New York, Churchill Livingstone, 1982, pp 121–136.
20. Watson WC, Sullivan SN: Hypertonicity of the cricopharyngeal sphincter; a cause of globus sensation. *Lancet* 1974;2:1417–1419.
21. Hunt PS, Connell AM, Smiley TB: The cricopharyngeal sphincter in gastric reflux. *Gut* 1970;11:303–306.
22. Stanciu C, Bennett JR: Upper esophageal yield pressures in normal subjects and patients with gastroesophageal reflux. *Thorax* 1974;29:459–462.
23. Gerhardt DC, Shock TJ, Bordeaux RA, et al: Human upper esophageal sphincter; response to volume, osmotic and acid stimuli. *Gastroenterology* 1978;75:268–274.
24. Hallewell JD, Cole TB: Isolated head and neck symptoms due to hiatus hernia. *Arch Otolaryngol* 1970;92:499–501.
25. Kilman WJ, Goyal RK: Disorders of pharyngeal and upper esophageal sphincter motor function. *Arch Intern Med* 1976;136:592–601.
26. Hurwitz AL, Nelson JA, Haddad JK: Oropharyngeal dysphagia. Manometric and cineradiographic esophagraphic findings. *Am J Dig Dis* 1975;20:313–324.
27. Reichert TJ, Bluestone CD, Stool SE, et al: Congenital cricopharyngeal achalasia. *Ann Otol Rhinol Laryngol* 1977;86:603–610.
28. Roed-Petersen K: The pharyngoesophageal sphincter. *Dan Med Bull* 1979;26:275–281.
29. Riley CM: Familial dysautonomia. *Adv Pediatr* 1957;5:157–190.
30. Marguilies SI, Bruut PW, Donner MW, et al: Familial dysautonomia, a cineradiographic study of the swallowing mechanism. *Radiology* 1968;90:107–112.
31. Ellis FH, Schlegel JF, Lynch VP, et al: Cricopharyngeal myotomy for pharyngo-esophageal diverticulum. *Ann Surg* 1969;170:340–349.
32. Duranceau A, Rheault MJ, Jamieson GG: Physiologic response to cricopharyngeal myotomy and diverticulum suspension. *Surgery* 1983;94:655–662.

CHAPTER 15

Gastroesophageal
Reflux and pH Testing

Wallace C. Wu, MB, BS

Gastroesophageal reflux disease (GERD), with its complications, is one of the most common diseases seen by the gastroenterologist. A survey of normal control subjects showed that 7% experienced heartburn daily, 14% at least weekly, and 15% at least monthly.[1] Therefore, in that particular study, 36% of the surveyed population had symptoms of GERD at least once a month. Testing for GERD has been reviewed extensively elsewhere[2]; in this chapter we will concentrate on the role of esophageal manometry and the use of intraesophageal pH probe in the evaluation of patients with suspected GERD.

ESOPHAGEAL MANOMETRY

The role of esophageal manometry as a diagnostic test in GERD is somewhat limited (see Chapter 1). In summary, patients with GERD, as a group, tend to have decreased lower esophageal sphincter (LES) pressure[3] and lower peristaltic amplitude[3,4] in the esophageal body. However, the presence of these motility findings by themselves are not diagnostic of GERD, since there is a large overlap with normal subjects. Esophageal manometry, therefore, is indicated only when the diagnosis of GERD is in doubt; the finding of very low LES pressure ($<$ 6 mm Hg) will support this diagnosis. It should also be performed prior to antireflux surgery, since the presence of a significant motility disorder may be a relative contraindication to surgery.

INTRAESOPHAGEAL pH MEASUREMENTS

Since GERD involves the reflux of acidic gastric contents into the esophagus, the pH probe has been used in various ways as a diagnostic tool. At present, most of the older tests using the pH probe, such as the standard acid-reflux test and acid-clearance test, have been superseded by continuous ambulatory pH monitoring.

Standard Acid-Reflux Test

The standard acid-reflux test (SART) utilizes short-term intraesophageal pH monitoring. This, of course, should test the competency of the antireflux barrier. A pH probe is placed 5 cm above the proximal margin of the manometrically determined LES. Reflux is first tested in the resting supine position. The patient is then turned to the right and left lateral and 20° head-down positions. During each position, the patient is asked to breathe normally, breathe deeply, perform Valsalva and Mueller maneuvers, and cough. A reflux episode is defined as a drop in pH to less than 4. Then 300 cc of 0.1N HCl will be instilled into the stomach and the above maneuvers repeated.[5] It is assumed that patients who reflux at rest will have more severe GERD than patients who reflux only upon stress. The basal SART was said to have a sensitivity of 40% and a specificity of 99%, whereas the SART with loading has a sensitivity of 84% and a specificity of 83%.[6] Unfortunately, there has never been any agreement as to the best way to perform or to interpret this test, and the advent of ambulatory monitoring made the performance of this test redundant.

Acid-Clearance Test

The acid-clearance test (ACT) was first described by Booth et al.[7] This test also involves placing the pH probe 5 cm above the LES. Fifteen cubic centimeters of 0.1N HCl are then infused into the esophagus. The patient is instructed to swallow at 30-sec intervals. The acid-clearance time is defined as the number of swallows required to elevate the intraesophageal pH to above 5. Normal subjects can clear the esophagus in approximately 10–12 swallows. Unfortunately, the results of this test tend to vary even on different days in the same subjects. Also, as many as 50% of reflux patients may have a normal test. At this time, this test is only of research interest.

Prolonged Intraesophageal pH Monitoring

In 1969, Spencer first reported the use of the pH probe for continuous prolonged monitoring of esophageal pH for 18 hours.[8] This was followed in 1974 by the landmark study of Johnson and DeMeester.[9] They established 24-hour esophageal pH monitoring as a clinically effective tool in the diagnosis of GERD. Their technique utilizes the Beckman pH probe placed transnasally 5 cm above the LES, as defined by manometry. A reference electrode is required and attached to the forearm. These are connected to a standard pH meter and recorder that are housed on a movable cart. This set-up allows the patient some freedom of movement, but the patient must be hospitalized for the study. The patient also is on a restricted diet that contains no substance with pH less than 5. The study is, therefore, conducted in as near-physiological condition as possible. Reflux is defined as a drop in pH to less than 4. The number and the length of reflux episodes are noted. Johnson and DeMeester used six different criteria in their studies to define gastroesophageal (GE) reflux. These parameters are still being used. Table 15.1 lists these six parameters with values for normal subjects in their laboratory. Also included are values for normal subjects obtained during ambulatory monitoring in our laboratory. These are not significantly different from the normal values obtained by Johnson and DeMeester with in-hospital testing.

Johnson and DeMeester established the usefulness of 24-hour esophageal pH monitoring as a research and clinical tool in GERD. It is now accepted that the sensitivity of prolonged pH monitoring is 88% with a specificity of 98%.[6] Although widely accepted, this test was never widely used, since the patient needs to be hospitalized and the equipment needed for the performance of this test is somewhat cumbersome. This test is presently being replaced by ambulatory pH monitoring.

Ambulatory Intraesophageal pH Monitoring

The past few years have seen the advent of many commercially available systems using microcomputer-based data collection and analysis devices. This allows the studies to be performed on a purely ambulatory basis (Fig. 15.1), removing the need for hospitalization of the patients.[10] The advent of computer technology also enables data to be analyzed in a more efficient fashion. As indicated in Table 15.1, the normals obtained with the ambulatory system are not significantly different from the normals obtained by Johnson and DeMeester.

TABLE 15.1 Normal Values for 24-Hour pH Monitoring

	Johnson and DeMeester[9] (N = 15)		Bowman Gray School of Medicine[10] (N = 20)	
	$\bar{x} \pm 1$ SD	Upper Limits of Normal ($\bar{x} + 2$ SD)	$\bar{x} \pm 1$ SD	Upper Limits of Normal ($\bar{x} + 2$ SD)
Percent of time pH < 4				
Total	1.478% ± 1.381%	<4.2%	1.27% ± 1.56	<4.4%
Recumbent	0.286% ± 0.467%	<1.2%	0.35% ± 0.73	<1.8%
Upright	2.33% ± 1.975%	<6.3%	1.71% ± 2.07	<5.9%
Number of total episodes	20.6 ± 14.773	<50	18.30 ± 16.40	<51
Number of episodes ≥ 5 min	0.6 ± 1.241	≤3	0.7 ± 1.69	≤4
Longest episode	2.866 min ± 2.689 min	<9.2 min		
Recumbent			1.11 min ± 2.25 min	<5.6
Upright			4.19 min ± 6.29 min	<16.8

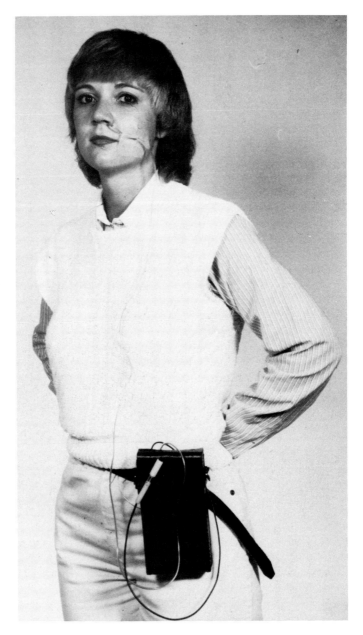

FIGURE 15.1 Normal volunteer with an ambulatory pH monitoring system.

There are six commercial ambulatory monitoring systems available in the United States at this time. Although their durability is still open to questions, all of them are adequate for routine clinical usage. At this point, the major unresolved issue concerning equipment is what kind of electrodes should be used (Fig. 15.2). The choices are the telemetric capsule or glass and antimony electrodes. Combined-glass electrodes, which incorporate a reference lead in the bulb, are also now commercially available in the United States. The capsule and the combined-glass electrode do not require the use of a reference lead. Hence, errors relating to problems with reference electrodes do not occur. This is the major advantage with both the combined glass electrode and the capsule, as compared with the standard glass and antimony electrodes.

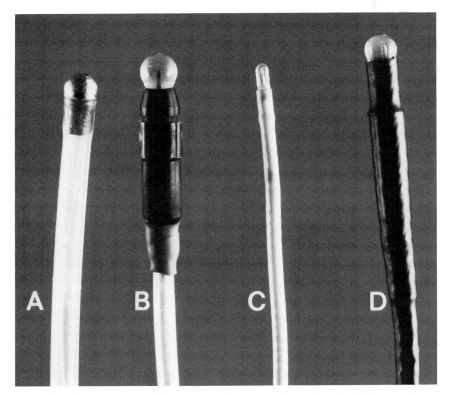

FIGURE 15.2 Different types of pH electrodes that are available: (A) Sandhill P32 pH antimony electrode; (B) Radiometer GK2803C combined-glass electrode; (C) Microelectrode MI-506 small-caliber glass electrode (particularly useful in pediatric patients); (D) Beckman 39042 glass electrode. All except B need a reference electrode.

By convention, the pH probe is placed 5 cm above the manometrically defined LES. This naturally implies that one cannot place a pH probe without an esophageal motility laboratory. Other methods of placement of the probe have been investigated. These include either using measurements obtained at endoscopy or noting the level at which the pH drops below 4 on insertion of the probe. These two measurements have been compared with the measurements obtained by esophageal manometry.[11] The results of this preliminary study indicate that measurements based on the pH change or endoscopy are not accurate enough for placement. Other studies have shown that placement of the probe at different levels in the esophagus will record different amounts of GE reflux.[12] Therefore, at this time, it seems clear that pH probes for 24-hour pH monitoring should preferably be placed manometrically.

The ideal period of time required for monitoring is also not settled. Most authors perform the study over a 24-hour period. However, studies for 3 hours postprandially or for a total of 8 and 12 hours have all been performed and reported.[13-16] Since postprandial and nocturnal reflux may both be important features in GERD, the period of monitoring should theoretically include at least a postprandial and a nocturnal supine period. Thus, it appears that the minimum amount of time required for monitoring should be 12 hours.

The interpretation of the 24-hour pH recording still remains somewhat controversial. Johnson had proposed a composite 24-hour pH reflux score in addition to the six parameters listed in Table 15.1.[9] The use of the score increased the sensitivity to 84%, as compared to 82% and 78% for percentage time pH less than 4 in the recumbent and total periods respectively. In our experience, we have found that it may be extremely difficult to define specific "reflux episodes" on a tracing, as shown in Figure 15.3. Hence, we have suggested that the major criteria that should be used are the total percentage time pH less than 4 over the entire 24-hour period and in the upright and supine positions. The 24-hour intraesophageal pH study is also an endogenous Bernstein test (Figs. 15.4, 15.5). Additional information may be obtained by specifically relating the spontaneous occurrence of the patient's symptoms with reflux episodes. Therefore, we have recently proposed that the symptoms experienced during the monitored period should be incorporated in the interpretation of the tracing.[10] This approach is still being evaluated at this time.[17]

Clearly, 24-hour pH monitoring is not needed in all patients with GERD. We suggest the following clinical indications: (1) patients with atypical presentations, such as pulmonary or ENT manifestations; (2) selected patients with noncardiac chest pain; (3) patients with typical symptoms but other negative diagnostic studies for GERD; and (4) assessment of patients before and after antireflux surgery.

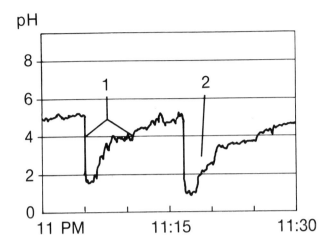

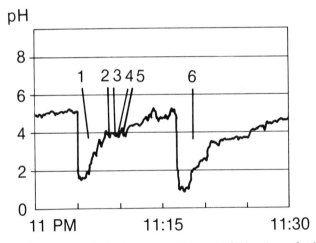

FIGURE 15.3 Varying numbers of episodes depending on the definition chosen for the end of a reflux episode.

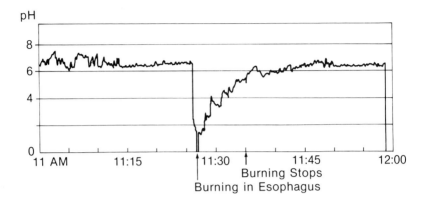

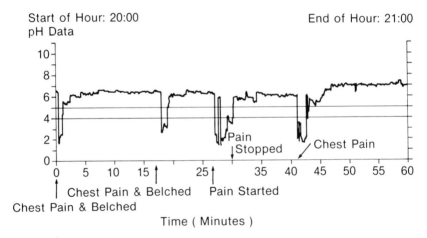

FIGURE 15.4 Two patients reporting symptoms with good correlation with pH activity.

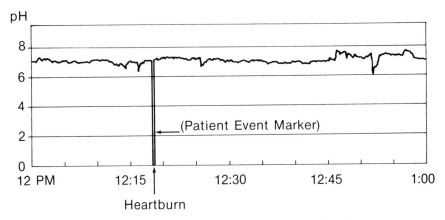

FIGURE 15.5 Patient reporting heartburn with no correlation with pH activity.

REFERENCES

1. Nebel OT, Fornes MF, Castell DO: Symptomatic gastroesophageal reflux incidence and precipitating factors. *Am J Dig Dis* 1976;21:953–956.
2. Castell DO, Wu WC, Ott DJ: *Gastroesophageal Reflux Disease. Pathogenesis, Diagnosis, Therapy.* New York, Futura Publishing, 1985.
3. Knuff TE, Benjamin SB, Worsham F, et al: Histologic evaluation of chronic gastroesophageal reflux: an evaluation of biopsy methods and diagnostic criteria. *Dig Dis Sci* 1984;29:194–201.
4. Kahrilas PJ, Dodds WJ, Hogan WJ, et al: Esophageal peristaltic dysfunction in peptic esophagitis. *Gastroenterology* 1986;91:897–904.
5. Kantrowitz PA, Corson JG, Fleischli DJ, et al: Measurement of gastroesophageal reflux. *Gastroenterology* 1968;56:666–673.
6. Richter JE, Castell DO: Gastroesophageal reflux. Pathogenesis, diagnosis, and therapy. *Ann Int Med* 1982;97:93–103.
7. Booth DG, Kemmerer WI, Skinner DB: Acid clearing from the distal esophagus. *Arch Surg* 1968;96:731–734.
8. Spencer J: Prolonged pH recording in the study of gastro-oesophageal reflux. *Br J Surg* 1969;56:912–914.
9. Johnson LF, DeMeester TR: Twenty-four-hour pH monitoring of the distal esophagus: a quantitative measure of gastroesophageal reflux. *Am J Gastroenterol* 1974;62:325–332.
10. Ward BW, Wu WC, Richter JE, et al: Ambulatory 24-hour esophageal pH monitoring. Technology searching for a clinical application. *J Clin Gastroenterol* 1986;8(suppl 1):59–67.
11. Walther B, DeMeester TR: Placement of the esophageal pH electrode for 24-hour esophageal pH monitoring, in DeMeester TR, Skinner DB (eds): *Esophageal Disorders.* New York, Raven Press, 1985, pp 539–541.
12. Johansson KE, Tibbling L: Evaluation of the 24-hour pH test at two different levels of the esophagus, in DeMeester TR, Skinner DB (eds): *Esophageal Disorders.* New York, Raven Press, 1985, pp 579–582.

13. Fink SM, McCallum RW: The role of prolonged esophageal pH monitoring in the diagnosis of gastroesophageal reflux. *JAMA* 1984;252:1160–1164.
14. Rokkas T, Anggiansah A, Uzoechina E, et al: The role of shorter than 24-h pH monitoring periods in the diagnosis of gastro-oesophageal reflux. *Scand J Gastroenterol* 1986;21:614–620.
15. Choiniere L, Miller L, Ilves R, et al: Comparison of 8-hour studies with 24-hour studies, in DeMeester TR, Skinner DB (eds): *Esophageal Disorders.* New York, Raven Press, 1985, pp 583–588.
16. Walther B, DeMeester TR: Comparison of 8- and 16-hour esophageal pH monitoring, in DeMeester TR, Skinner DB (eds): *Esophageal Disorders.* New York, Raven Press, 1985, pp 589–591.
17. Wiener GJ, Copper JB, Wu WC, et al: The symptom index (SI): an endogenous 24-hour provocative test for symptoms of gastroesophageal reflux (GER). *Gastroenterology* 1987;92:1694.

Index

A

Abnormal contractions, 121–128
  of esophageal body, 71–76
Abnormal motor responses, 85–88
Achalasia, 107
  atypical findings in, 112–114
  clinical presentation of, 107–108
  endoscopic features of, 108
  esophageal body assessment in, 110–112
  LES relaxation testing in, 109–110
  manometric findings in, 109
  radiologic features in, 108
  treatment of, 115–117
Acid-clearance test, 199
Acid-perfusion test, 143, 147; *see also*
      Bernstein test
Aging, 178
Alcohol, effects on esophageal motility,
  157–158
Ambulatory intraesophageal pH monitoring,
  152–153, 200–207
Amyloidosis, 169, 172
Amyotrophic lateral sclerosis, 176
Anorexia nervosa, 10
Aperistalsis, 114
Atropine, 25, 57

B

Balloon distension, 151–152
Barium studies, 144
Bechet's syndrome, 168
Bernstein test, 56

C

Calcium channel-blocking agents, 22
Calibration of equipment, 35–36
Cardiac disease, 144
Cardiospasm, 108
Central nervous system, involuntary
  responses of, 14–16
Central nervous system lymphoma, 176
Cerebrovascular disease, 176
Chagas' disease, 178
Chest pain, 57, 108, 118–119, 130, 134
Chest pain syndrome, 9
Chronic idiopathic intestinal
  pseudo-obstruction, 176–177
Collagen-vascular diseases, 163–165
Computer analysis
  LES pressure and relaxation, 100–102
  peristaltic wave parameters by, 97–100
  UES pressure and relaxation, 102–103
Computer applications, in esophageal
  pressure profiling, 91–103
Contraction amplitude, 66–67, 81–83
Coronary angiography, 144
Cricopharyngeal achalasia, 195

D

Database, esophageal motility, 89; *see also*
  Computer analysis
Deglutitive inhibition, 18, 20
Dent sleeve, 5, 190
Dermatomyositis, 165
Diabetes mellitus, 168–169

Diffuse esophageal spasm, 88, 118
 historical background, 118–120
 LES pressure and relaxation in, 125–128
 manometric diagnosis of, 121–128
 pathophysiology and etiology of, 119
 symptoms of, 119–121
Diffuse motility disorder, 10
Distal esophageal amplitude, 67
 effect of age on, 81–82
Distal esophageal duration, effect of age on, 84
Distal esophageal velocity, 84
Duration response, 25–26
Dysphagia, 8, 107, 119, 173

E
Echocardiography, 144
Edrophonium (tensilon) test, 56–57, 147–149
Emotional stress, 107, 119
Endocrine disorders, 168–169
Endoscopy, 144
Esophageal baseline, 67–68
Esophageal body
 abnormal contractions, 71–76
 achalasia assessment and, 110
 amplitude, 66
 duration, 67–68
 velocity, 69
Esophageal manometry
 clinical applications of, 7–11
 computer applications in, 91–94
 diagnostic test in GERD, 198
 evaluation of GERD, 198
 evaluation of noncardiac chest pain, 145
 experience with healthy volunteers, 80–89
 historical overview, 3, 79–80
 in achalasia, 109
 in diagnosis of diffuse esophageal spasm, 121–128
 in UES, 192–193
 laboratory equipment and materials, 28–34
 pharyngoesophageal junction evaluation by, 190–193
 secondary motility disorder evaluation by, 163–180
 techniques in, 4–6
 use of, 6–7
 versus provocative testing, 149–151
Esophageal manometry catheter, 28
Esophageal motility, 156–159
Esophageal motility database, 89
Esophageal motility dysfunction, 7
Esophageal squeeze, 6

Esophageal symptoms, 8–10
Esophagus
 anatomy and physiology of, 13–18
 effect of aging on, 178–180
 exogenous factors affecting motility of, 156
 peristaltic control of, 24
 role of sphincters in, 19–24
 stages of swallowing in, 14–16

F
Food impaction, 121
Food quality, effect on esophageal function, 158–159

G
Gallbladder study, 144
Gastric air bubble, 108
Gastric baseline, 39, 61
Gastric cancer, 144
Gastric pressure, 20
Gastrin, 3
Gastroesophageal (GE) reflux, 6, 9, 22, 108
Gastroesophageal reflux disease (GERD), 156
 manometric evaluation of, 198
 pH testing of, 199–207

H
Heartburn, 108
High-amplitude esophageal contractions, 6
High-pressure zone, 183
Hypercontracting sphincter, 139
Hypopharynx, 184–185

I
Infusion rate, 4
Intraesophageal peristaltic activity, 4
 pressure measurements, 6
Intraesophageal pressure transducers, 79, 121
Intragastric pressure, 20
Intubation, 37–39
Involuntary responses, 14–16

L
Latency gradient, 25
Low-compliance pneumohydraulic infusion, 79, 121
Lower esophageal sphincter (LES)
 effect of alcohol on, 157–158
 effect of food on, 158–159
 effect of smoking on, 156–157
 hormonal control of, 22
 physiologic functions of, 21–22
 pressure changes in, 22–24, 100–102
 pressure measurements, 5–6, 61–66, 85

relaxation in, 20–23, 42–47, 62,
    109–110, 125–128
temperature effects on, 159–161
Lubrication, 37

M

Manometric study, 60
    equipment calibration, 35
    esophagus evaluation by, 48–55
    final reporting of, 78
    intubation, 37–39
    LES pressure measurements, 42–48
    motility recordings, 39
    patient preparation for, 35–39
    provocative testing, 56–57
    UES pressure measurements, 57–59
Metabolic disorders, 168–169
Mixed connective tissue disease, 165
Multiple sclerosis, 174–175
Myasthenia gravis, 174
Myenteric plexus, 25
Myotonic dystrophy, 173

N

Neuromuscular disorders, 172–176
Neuropathy, 168
Nocturnal regurgitation, 107
Noncardiac chest pain, 131, 143; *see also*
    Chest pain
    clinical experience with, 149–151
    esophageal manometric evaluation of, 145
    esophageal testing of, 144–145
    future developments for evaluation of,
        151–153
    initial evaluation of, 144
    nutcracker esophagus and, 145–146
    provocative testing for, 146–151
Nonspecific esophageal motility disorders,
    79, 139–141
Nutcracker esophagus
    definition of, 131–136
    hypertensive LES and, 138–139
    noncardiac chest pain and, 145–146
    nonspecific motility disorders of, 139–141
    perspectives on, 136–138
    provocative testing of, 149

O

Off-response, 25
On-response, 25
Oropharyngeal dysphagia, 194

P

Pain threshold, 143, 149
Parkinson's disease, 175

Peptic stricture, 108
Peptic ulceration, 144
Perfusion techniques, 4
Peristalsis, 16–19, 52
Peristaltic clearing wave, 16
Peristaltic pressure, 4, 6
Peristaltic sequence, 6
Peristaltic wave parameters, 97–100
Pharmacologic stimulation, 143
Pharyngeal contractions, 77, 102–103, 173,
    187–189
pH testing, of gastroesophageal reflux
    disease, 199–207
Physiograph, 30
    calibration of, 35–36
Pneumatic dilatation, 115–116
Point of respiratory reversal, 43
Polymyositis, 165
Post-relaxation augmentation, 76
Pressure inversion point, 43
Pressure profiling, 91–103
Progressive systemic sclerosis (PSS), 164–167
Provocative tests, 10, 56–57
    acid-perfusion, 147
    edrophonium, 147–149
    historical perspectives, 146–147
    in noncardiac chest pain, 146–151
    of nutcracker esophagus, 149
    versus esophageal manometry, 149–151

R

Radionuclide transit studies, 108
Rapid pull-through (RPT) technique, 5, 42,
    61, 100–101, 184
Rapid sequential swallowing, 18
Reflux esophagitis, 144
Rheumatoid arthritis, 166
Riley-Day syndrome, 195

S

Secondary esophageal motility disorders
    aging and, 178–180
    Chagas', 178
    chronic idiopathic intestinal
        pseudo-obstruction, 176–177
    collagen-vascular, 163–165
    endocrine and metabolic, 168–169
    neuromuscular, 172–176
Sjögren's syndrome, 168
Sphincter pressure, 4–5
Standard acid-reflux test, 199
Station pull-through (SPT) technique, 5, 43,
    62, 101, 184
Swallowing, stages of, 14–16

T

Temperature effects, on esophageal
    function, 159–161
Tetrodotoxin, 22, 25
Thyroid disease, 169
Tobacco-containing products, effects on
    esophageal motility, 156–157
Tonic closure, 22

U

Upper esophageal sphincter (UES), 13, 20,
    183
  disorders of, 193–196
  hypertensive, 193
  hypopharynx coordination with, 185–189
  hypotensive, 195

manometric assessment of, 192–193
pharyngeal contractions and, 77
pressure measurements, 57–58, 76–77,
    100–102, 184
relaxation, 76, 185–188, 195–196

V

Vasoactive intestinal polypeptide, 22

W

Water-filled catheters, 3
Water-infusion system, 28
Weight loss, 107
Wet swallow, 6

Y

Yield pressure, 4